D1146190

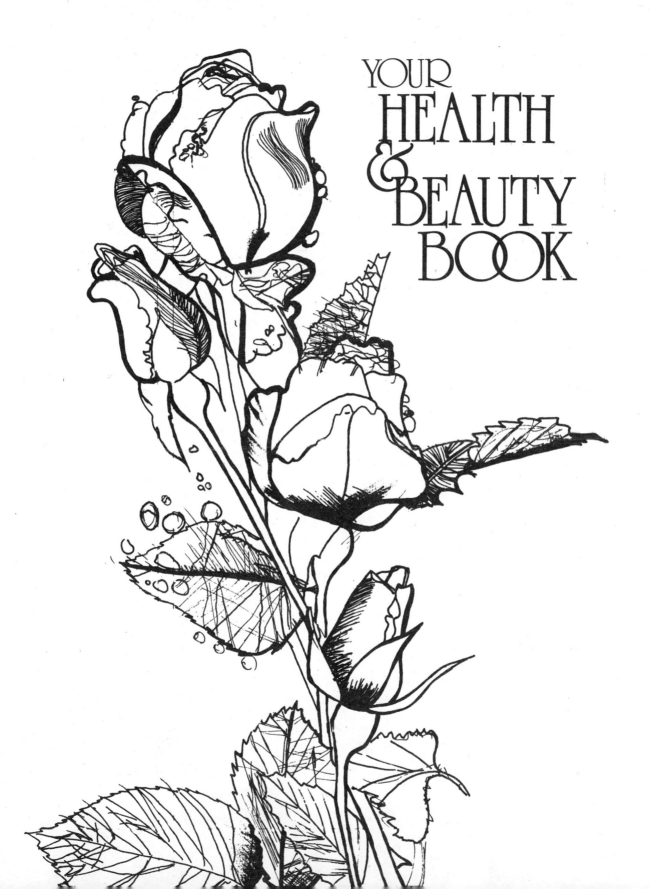

YOUR
HEALTH
&
BEAUTY
BOOK

Clare Maxwell-Hudson has also written

KALEIDOSCOPE OF BEAUTY (Octagon Press, 1968)
THE NATURAL BEAUTY BOOK (Macdonald and Jane's, 1976)

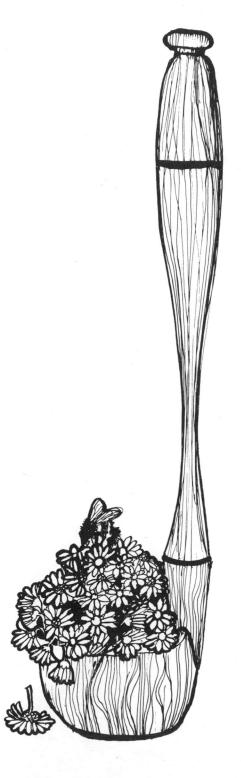

YOUR HEALTH & BEAUTY BOOK

Make your home into a health farm

CLARE MAXWELL-HUDSON

Illustrations by Janina Ede

MACDONALD GENERAL BOOKS
MACDONALD AND JANE'S
LONDON AND SYDNEY

First published in 1979 by Macdonald General Books,
Macdonald and Jane's Publishers Limited,
Paulton House, 8 Shepherdess Walk,
London, N.1

Copyright in the text © Clare Maxwell-Hudson, 1979
Copyright in the illustrations © Macdonald and Jane's, 1979

ISBN 0 354 04410 2

Phototypeset by
MS Filmsetting Limited,
Frome, Somerset

Printed in Great Britain by
Purnell & Sons Limited,
Paulton (Bristol) and London.

Contents

AUTHOR'S ACKNOWLEDGEMENTS

My most grateful thanks for all their encouragement and advice are
offered to:
Annette Lawrence, MAHE, for all her help on the *Diet* section;
Bella Wood, for all her help on the *Exercise* and *Massage* sections;
Robin Price of the Wellcome Library, for checking some of my facts;
Gill Stewart, for typing and her general enthusiasm for the material;
Mina, Miles and Pat Williams, for their help, advice and encouragement;
Susan Fleming, for her work on the manuscript;
Janine Ede, for her wonderful illustrations;
Margaret Kilrenny, for all her help;
and to all my beautiful clients for being such willing guinea pigs in my
experiments; without their help through the years, this book could never
have been written.

TO GILBERTE BRUNSDON-LENAERTS
in gratitude

Introduction

Beauty, they say, is in the eye of the beholder. But I think it is even more in the attitude of the person beheld! For if you are to be successfully beautiful, you *must* have confidence. I have met and been consulted by so many men and women who feel that their looks have deteriorated, or that they are in a rut – when, in fact, they were simply not making the most of themselves.

If you feel that you fall into this category too, do not despair. Now is the time to start to do something about yourself. There is no reason why every one of us should not look and feel both healthy and attractive.

There are, however, so many books about health and beauty written at the moment, that you may be confused about the conflicting claims and theories. For this reason, you will probably want to know what you are going to find in the pages here.

What I have tried to do is write a *practical* guide to health and beauty, with clearly laid-out instructions on what to do and how to do it. In other words, how to turn your home into your own, easily organized, health and beauty farm. I have included nothing that my clients and I have not tried and tested.

Essentially, I have tried to answer the question: how can one become, and remain, healthy and attractive? I chose the title because it is simple. And all the way through the book, I have tried to make everything as straightforward and simple as possible. My basic attitude is that health is the natural spring-board to beauty. And that a balanced basis of health *and* beauty results in poise and self-confidence.

I can really promise you that all it takes is a little effort on your part. Over the years I have helped a great number of people, and I can help you – but I do need a little cooperation.

Did you know that a woman's skin often improves with age? That the skin of a thirty-year-old can be better than that of a teenager? Chronological age is not important – someone of seventy years of age can be healthier than another person of forty. Every woman knows that 'if you feel good, you look good'. This kind of information (and there is a lot of it throughout this book), is introduced for the very definite purpose of pointing out the vital fact that what counts more than anything in beauty and health is *attitude*.

Whether you are young or not-so-young, whether you have perfect features or not, always remember to be yourself. As Francis Bacon said: 'There is no perfect beauty that hath not some strangeness in proportion.' So we begin your health and beauty course by affirming the positive, as well as the personal, approach.

Books on beauty and slimming so often approach their subject in terms of waging battle and suffering. The practising beautician, therefore, finds that before she can release the inward beauty of her client, she has to help her readjust from this misery and replace it with a more constructive approach.

To bridge the gap, as I have discovered during many years of experience, is a matter of manner and method. So, don't try to be a martyr, or full of grim determination: I only need that degree of cooperation which will make more of your looks and help you project yourself better.

Let us unlock some of the hang-ups by a simple change of focus which I have used with success in more cases than I can count. First, reclaim for yourself the concept that it is everyone's right to be attractive. There is far too much guilt and defensiveness about all this. One does not have to be a woman's-libber to be aware that if a man looks at an oil painting, it is regarded as an aesthetic experience; but if a woman looks at a beautifully designed dress or piece of jewellery, or a health and beauty process – this is counted as frivolous. Once you get this into perspective, you will see that there is really no difference. 'Cultivate your person,' said Confucius. And by making yourself look better and feel better, you will be making a great difference to the lives of others as well.

So don't be defensive or aggressive. But you must promise me at least some attention. I know that you are busy: almost everyone is. But there are 168 hours in every week (of which 119 are waking hours), and I am asking you to set aside a very small proportion of this time. You will be surprised how easy – and how inexpensive – it is.

We all want to look and feel good, but most of us don't know how to go about it. Or more accurately, we neglect to do anything about ourselves, and then wonder why we don't look our best. What is *your* best? Let me help you to find out. Let us go through the entire book together, and see in what way you can emerge from your dream. Let us make it reality together.

However busy and hectic a life you lead, you can always manage to do something that you really *want* to do. And I hope that when you read this book you will want to try and follow the courses I have planned for you. Time is elastic: the more you have to do, the more you are able to do.

I have started with a Two-Day Blitz, which is exactly what it says – two days of attacking yourself on all fronts: diet, exercise, massage and pampering. Within forty-eight hours you should experience a lightening effect, which will leave you feeling infinitely healthier.

Feeling so good after just two days will, I hope, encourage you to continue on to the Seven-Day Campaign. During this week I ask you to give yourself at least an hour's worth of attention daily, and to go on our carefully planned diet.

After this I am assuming that you will feel so wonderful that you will want to maintain this new healthy you, and that you will easily go on the Three-Week Health Kick. On this I only expect you to give yourself a little time each day for the essentials: exercise (only 5 minutes!), washing and skin care. Everything else can be fitted in when you have the time.

Start off with *enthusiasm*, and keep that enthusiasm all the time. It will certainly pay off when you look at yourself in the cold light of reason, and in the rôle of your sternest critic. For we cannot ever really deceive ourselves, can we? If we are looking good, and once we honestly know it, this knowledge quickly communicates to others. All our labours will not have been in vain.

I cannot stress too much the fact that it is entirely up to you to make yourself more attractive; someone the beholder cannot help but admire.

Obviously any book on health and beauty must go into the subject of diet. I find this a fascinating subject, and so have included a section on nutrition, as well as giving you hints on diets and how to keep to them. For good nutrition – a good diet – is synonymous with health.

Being a great believer in the benefits of massage I have included a chapter on why you need it and how to massage. (In fact I wrote so much about it that the type face for this book had to be set smaller to fit it all in!)

I cannot stress enough the importance of skin care. I go into this very thoroughly, and show you step by step how to make your own cosmetics. Also, believing as I do that hair is one of the greatest of personal adornments, I have given recipes for hair conditioners and rinses, many of which I have collected myself from all parts of the world. From the African continent, through Turkey and Persia to the plains and mountains of Central Asia, I have been able to indulge my love of travel, while searching for beauty items. And I've been lucky enough to obtain, sometimes only by accident, other times by sheer force of questioning, many most delightful concoctions and salves.

Finally, no book on health would be complete without a section on exercise. Exercise can be fun and I have made every attempt to make this chapter as light and easy as possible.

Throughout the book I have jotted down ideas and hints that my clients and I find useful or amusing. I have pointed out the way to make your bathroom a sanctuary, how to create your own bath oils and pot-pourris, the virtues of drinking a lot of water, of having plenty of fresh air, and the importance of relaxation and sleep.

In the field of beauty, doing something about yourself means giving yourself the right amount of time and the correct proportion of routine: using, in fact, variety and stability (the essentials of a happy life), to guide your programme of bringing out the very best in you.

I have therefore built into this book the procedures which should help you avoid too much routine, and included the right amount of change – too much can make people frantic!

Before you do a single thing I recommend (and everything has been very carefully worked out and tested) I want you to start to look around you. Tests have shown that people who look optimistic are thought to be more attractive than those who do not smile or laugh. As Idries Shah says in *Learning How to Learn* (Octagon Press, 1978): 'If you cannot laugh frequently and genuinely, you have no soul.' And have you noticed how often, referring to beautiful women, poets and others speak of their attractiveness as being a form of happiness as from 'the inward soul'? *To enjoy life is also to improve your own image of yourself.*

Imagine that you are beautiful, fascinating, slim and madly attractive – and you will be amazed to find that others will feel the same about you!

In fact, an experiment of this kind was carried out a few years ago in the psychology department of an American university. The professor asked his students to treat a very shy and rather plain member of the class as if she was the most attractive and popular girl on the campus. And do you know . . . by the end of that very term she *was*!

You don't have to believe me. Just try it out for yourself. Don't tell anyone, but really concentrate for just one day, telling yourself that you look marvellous: and wait for the compliments! I am convinced that this is one of the reasons why so many French women look so attractive. From their childhood they are told that they are beautiful, and this seems to give them a confidence that shines through.

Test the theory in another way, rather like that psychological experiment. Tell someone that she is attractive, and you will not have to wait long for a subtle change in appearance that tells you that it is working.

Anxiety has the opposite effect. If you think that you look fat, ugly and generally unattractive, then you *will* look so. *Don't!*

'*A sense of health, intelligence and quirky imperfections lend a reality and express individuality. Women who make a personal statement with their façade seem more interesting. They can never have beauty unless they believe in it*' (Kenneth of New York).

And don't tell yourself that you are too busy! I am assuming that you *are* busy: that you are often tired; that you may have to do exercises while the kettle is boiling, or massage yourself while the baby is asleep; that you may have to fit in a shampoo when you get home from work. But remember, this course has already been carried out successfully by many, many people in about the same situation as you: people living a full life, crowded with responsibilities. I am certain that, like them, if you stick to my carefully planned programme, the results will make your effort well worth while.

My system of health and beauty starts where every female instinctively begins when she knows she is not making the most of herself. And the best beauty therapy consists of an inherent understanding married with correct technique. It really brings success.

Beauty is not what current fashion designates as beauty. Extremes were always with us and always will be, as long as there is someone left on this planet to read books on fashion. In my opinion, what has more to do with beauty than anything else is attitude of mind. That, coupled with true good health, will make a swan out of the plainest duckling.

Good luck!

Clare Maxwell-Hudson, April 1979

'Saints and Kings, Prophets and Dervishes all bow down before beauty descending from the unknown world.
'We love beauty because it is not merely of this earth: beauty in the human being is a reflection of celestial beauty itself.'

Mahmud Shabistari, *Secret Garden*, Sufi Writings of the 13th century.

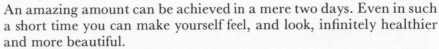

The Two-Day Blitz

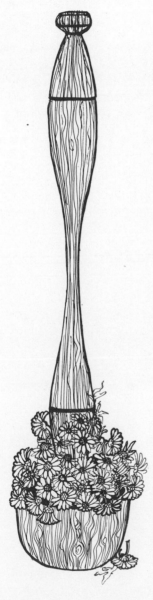

An amazing amount can be achieved in a mere two days. Even in such a short time you can make yourself feel, and look, infinitely healthier and more beautiful.

This is the perfect thing to do if you are going away on holiday and none of your clothes fit; if you are just recovering from a Christmas of over-eating and over-drinking; or, if you just feel you need to take yourself in hand. It's almost miraculous how two days can make you feel and look slimmer and totally relaxed and refreshed.

Don't be put off by the fact that you will be on liquids only. I used to think that people who managed to fast must be incredibly strong-willed – which I am not. I really never imagined that I would either go on one, or if I did, manage to stick to it. But it's easy – and even enjoyable. I find the trick with going on a semi-fast, and in fact all dieting, is to convince yourself beforehand that you *really* want to do it – then it's easy and enjoyable. I can honestly say that while I was writing (and practising!) the *Two-day blitz*, I never once felt any pangs of hunger.

So before you start, really convince yourself that you want to go on it, and then it will be fun. It is worth it, you feel so marvellous afterwards.

This two-day blitz is useful for everyone, whether you wish to lose weight or not. If you are the right weight, it will simply make you feel cleaner, fresher and infinitely healthier. If you are overweight, you can easily lose anything from 3 to 6 lbs, and that will encourage you to go on a proper diet.

Organize your two days carefully and, preferably, ask a friend to join you. The two-day blitz will be much more enjoyable if you can compare notes and progress with someone. Even if you don't see each other, the fact that someone else is also living on liquids is reassuring – and it brings out your competitive spirit which helps to prevent you giving up.

If you have children, ask your husband to look after them for the whole two days; at best it will be a novel experience for him and for them, and at least, it will show him what you have to put up with every day! Or if your partner in the two-day blitz is your husband (or wife), arrange for the children to stay with some willing friends.

It is very important to tell those with whom you live of your plans for the two days. A dinner or lunch party would be fatal to your blitz; and to have to entertain and cook meals when you are starving yourself in the cause of health and beauty, can be demoralizing.

Throughout these two days you may drink as much water or herb tea as you like. Whenever you feel the pangs of hunger have a drink and they should go away – or at least diminish. Keep several bottles of mineral water in the refrigerator and a selection of herb teas all ready for use. The more liquid you drink the better.

I want you to try and avoid coffee and ordinary strong tea because they are stimulants and for these two days you are clearing, cleansing, detoxicating and purifying your system.

The day before

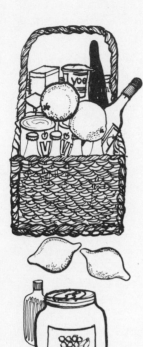

Make sure that you organize everything and everyone, so that for the next two days you are free to concentrate on yourself.

Pretend that you really are going to be away at a health farm with nothing to do but pamper yourself.

Make sure that you have the following:
Leotard, a large scarf, comfortable clothes and walking shoes, string glove or loofah, body lotion or almond oil, cleansing cream, cotton wool, skin tonic, rich massage cream, eyebrow tweezers, face pack (or an egg), moisturizer, manicure equipment (varnish remover, orange stick, emery board, hoof stick, cuticle cream, a buffer and varnish), tinfoil.

Shopping list
4 bottles mineral water
A variety of herbs to make teas (see page 31)
2 cans of vegetable juice or
    2 cans of consommé
Fruit juices (grape, unsweetened apple, and prune juice)
1 can tomato juice
1 small carton yoghurt (4–5 oz/100–125 g)
2 lemons, 2 oranges and 1 grapefruit
1 cucumber (to use for either drink or eyepads)
Eggs

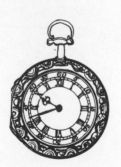

Ingredients needed for the recipes:

Mayonnaise face mask – 1 egg yolk, 1 tablespoon vinegar, ½ cup sunflower oil and 1 teaspoon honey.

Milk and honey bath oil – 2 eggs, ¼ cup sunflower oil, ¼ cup almond oil, 2 tablespoons honey, 2 teaspoons washing-up detergent, ¼ cup vodka and ½ cup milk.

Try and have an early night.

Day one

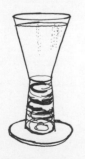

8.00 On waking go and get yourself a large glass of cold mineral water. Return to bed and read or relax while drinking it. The more water you drink today the better. Have a selection of different waters in the refrigerator, some still and some bubbly (with a little imagination it's just like drinking champagne!). All this water helps clear out your system and prevents you from feeling hungry.

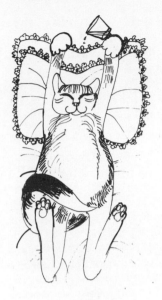

9.00   Stretch in bed. Imagine that you are a cat and really stretch your whole body.

1.   Stretch one side until it is completely taut, relax, and stretch the other side.
2.   Point your toes, pedal your feet, pushing the toes up and down. Relax the feet and wiggle them around and around.
3.   Lift your arms above your head and stretch each arm alternately. Feel the stretch going all the way down your side.
4.   Stretch the hand and fingers several times and then wiggle them around and around.

A final stretch of every part of your body and you should now be awake and ready to face the day.

9.15   **The mirror test**

Start by shocking yourself into action. Stand naked in front of a full-length mirror. Use a hand mirror as well (so that you can see your back view) and really look at yourself.

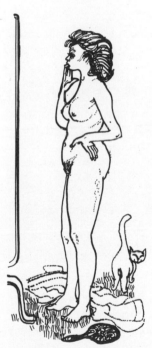

1.   Are you perfect?
2.   Would you be happy for the bitchiest person you know to see you now?
3.   Are you fit to be seen in a brief swimsuit on the beach? Really study your body. If you are plump and firm or tall and skinny and you are happy with your body then that's marvellous (we don't all have to look the same). You just want to find out your good points – and your bad points – so that you can make the best of yourself. A plump firm body is prettier than a slim flabby one, so be honest with yourself and don't be bullied by public opinion into trying to become something you are not. The only way you are ever going to look really beautiful is if *you* feel good. So it's up to you.

(a)   Note all your good points – write them down and remember to emphasize them.
(b)   Note all your bad points – and vow to improve them.
(c)   Write it all down. Fill in the charts at the back of the book. Go on – there are several charts so you can always rub it out later if it embarrasses you.
(d)   Measure yourself. Don't cheat and pull your tummy in – it's much more fun to be truthful and see your miraculous results.
(e)   Have you a photo of yourself that you really like? If so, even if it is ten years old, pin it up somewhere as a goal.

Last time I did the mirror test it was straight after an over-indulgent Christmas and I was so horrified at what I saw, that I took some photos of myself in my smallest bikini – and that really made me stick to the two-day blitz!

Weigh yourself

There are a few common figure faults, in both women and

men, which are largely a consequence of the way we live: the muscle tone in each of the areas – hips, tummy, upper-arms, waistline, thighs and bustline – is weak because normal every-day activity just isn't geared to giving it work to do. Even if your scales show a steady weight, the muscles may be slackening, and by a concentrated assault on the areas your mirror test has revealed as 'problem', you *can* achieve that firm lithe figure you dream of.

Bust. Every woman is different, obviously, but a droop in any size of breast is demoralizing and can look less than pretty.

Stomach. Does your stomach bulge even when you're holding it in? Is there any slack flesh?

Waistline. Can you find it?

Hips and buttocks. Is your hip measurement more than three inches bigger than your bust measurement (but make slight allowance for 'large bone structure'). Are your buttocks beginning to droop?

Thighs. Have you 'handles' on the outsides of your thighs, slack flesh on the inside?

Upper arms and shoulders. Can you grab more than an inch of 'slack' when you take the flesh between finger and thumb?

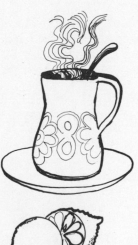

Firstly determine to do something about each and every one of the above faults you've found. And secondly, and most importantly, don't get depressed; they can all be corrected by diet, exercise and better posture. In each of these areas, bad habits may have to be changed permanently to ensure that the good results of your hard work last. Figure-faults do tend to keep returning – especially if you're in a job which involves sitting down for long periods (as most people are), stooping, or carrying heavy weights.

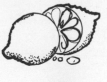

The purpose of this book is to try to help you to become, and stay, fitter, healthier and more beautiful.

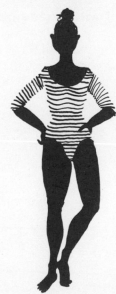

9.45   *Breakfast*. Hot lemon juice. Have a large mug of hot water and the juice of half a lemon. This is marvellously refreshing. If you find it too sour add a *small* teaspoon of honey to it.

10.00   Put on a leotard. I find leotards the most useful things when I am trying to slim. If I am feeling fat they show up all my bulges and goad me into staying on a diet – and when I am slim they make me feel so slinky and sylph-like that I want to remain like that, and so again keep me on the diet.

10.00   **Exercises** (pages 145–58)
Do the ten-minute warm-up routine to music; those are the

standing exercises. Today these exercises will probably take you longer than ten minutes because you are unfamiliar with the routine but once you know them they really will take that time or less. They are all very easy and enjoyable exercises. Then if you can manage it, do some of the floor exercises, concentrating on your problem areas.

After all that relax completely for five minutes by doing the relaxation exercises.

It's always much more fun to do exercises to music, so choose something with a strong beat and do your exercises by 'dancing' along with it.

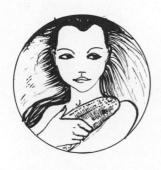

10.30 Scrub your body with a string glove (or loofah). This stimulates the skin and removes any roughness. If done every day it will greatly improve the texture of your skin, making it smooth and silky. Wash and apply some body lotion or almond oil. Wash, cleanse, tone and cream your face (see page 162) and then dress in comfortable clothes.

11.00 Have a cup of herb tea. On the two-day blitz we are detoxicating and purifying the system. There are numerous herbs and fruits which help this process, and so the juices I suggest are for this purpose. Fennel is a mild diuretic which helps remove impurities from the system, so why not try some fennel tea – it is delicious (see page 32).

11.30 Go outside and do some form of exercise. Go for a long energetic walk or for a bicycle ride. Or go swimming – but don't just float around lazily, really swim. Try and do at least ten lengths and if possible twenty! Breast stroke is good for the arms, bust and thighs. Backstroke and crawl exercise the back and legs. Or play tennis.

It doesn't really matter what you do, just be sure that you are getting some form of exercise, and preferably in the fresh air.

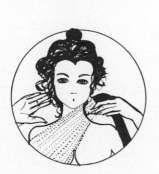

1.00 **After all that** energetic exercise you are probably feeling hot and sticky, so have a shower. Showers are quick and refreshing. Alternate the water from warm (never very hot) to cold – it makes one yelp but it is worth it because one feels so invigorated afterwards. If you don't have a shower, splash yourself to get the same enlivening effect. A shower is an instant pick-up.

1.30 *Lunch.* Have a glass of vegetable juice. Unless you have a juice extractor, I suggest that you use canned vegetable juice. There is a tremendous variety available and they are all delicious. Try a mixed vegetable juice or celery juice (which is said to clear the blood). Or have a bowl of consommé. Again it is such a long, complicated business making consommé that I suggest you have canned. It tastes delicious and is very low in calories.

1.45   *Relax.* Rest with your feet higher than your head. Read a light book, or you could even read about diets to get yourself into the mood!

2.30   **Body massage**
Massage makes one feel pampered, it relieves tension, stimulates the blood and nourishes, smoothes, softens and tones the skin. If practised strenuously enough, it can even maintain muscle tone, and break down fatty tissue. It is possible to massage yourself, but it is far easier, and more enjoyable, if you can exchange a body massage with a friend. You could do the massaging today and be massaged tomorrow (see *Massage* section, pages 81–112).

Start at your feet with the basic *stroking* movement, then work your way up your body to your shoulders and neck. Then be more drastic and *knead* your flesh as if you were kneading bread – again all over your body. Finish off by *clapping* and *slapping*, which is just what the words imply. A rhythmic, fast, bouncy movement here will stimulate the flow of blood to the veins. Use some almond oil to help in your massage or one of the creams in the *Massage* section.

3.30   Have a small glass of grape juice. Drink it for its purifying properties. At some health farms in Europe they give grape cures, where nothing but grapes are eaten, as it is claimed this is an effective treatment for obesity.

3.45   *Relax.* Either do nothing, or something you enjoy, but never have time to do. Sort out all your photos, or books. It is a marvellous time to reorganize your clothes. Try them on – if they are too tight put them at one end of the cupboard as a target.

4.30   Make up some cosmetics.
If I had to choose one beauty ingredient, I would choose eggs: they are so versatile, they can be used everywhere – on your face, on your hair and even in your bath.

We'll start by making mayonnaise. I suggest that you make this mayonnaise for several reasons. The first, because it is one of the very best face masks and does wonders for the skin; the second because it is absolutely marvellous as a hair conditioner (you can use the remains tomorrow before you wash your hair); and the third, because you almost undoubtedly have all the ingredients awaiting you in the kitchen.

1 egg yolk (if your hair is greasy or very fine, use the whole egg)
1 tablespoon cider vinegar
½ cup sunflower oil
1 teaspoon honey (optional)

Mix the egg, honey and vinegar together and then slowly, beating all the time, add in the oil. This mayonnaise contains all the necessary ingredients, eggs for nourishing, oil for lubricating and vinegar for its acidic value.

The milk and honey bath oil recipe that I give you tomorrow contains virtually the same ingredients and so you could easily make that up now as well (see page 27).

Both recipes are extremely easy and the results they give make them really well worth making.

5.00   Have some herb tea. Try peppermint tea or one of the mixtures I suggest on page 32.

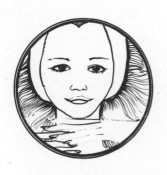

5.30   *Massage your face.* Or better still, swop a face massage with a friend. Already existing lines won't be magicked away, but massage can prevent the appearance of any more. As with the body, face massage tones up the muscles, and brings the blood to the surface. Gather together everything you need: cleansing cream, skin tonic, cotton wool, rich massage cream, eyebrow tweezers, your mayonnaise face mask, eye pads and moisturizer. (Use any of the creams and lotions recommended in the *Skin* section.)

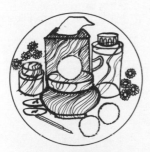

1.   First tie back your hair, but don't worry too much as you are washing it tomorrow.
2.   Apply a generous amount of cleansing cream and massage it in.
3.   Remove the cleansing cream with cotton wool that has been dampened with skin tonic.
4.   Massage the face. Remember always stroke upwards and outwards. Start at the base of the neck and stroke up the throat, then stroke outwards from the chin to the ears. Stroke upwards from the chin up by the nose to the forehead, then stroke around the eyes and on the forehead. See *Face massage* section, pages 108–111.
5.   Wipe any excess cream off with skin tonic.
6.   Tidy up your eyebrows.
7.   Steam your face.

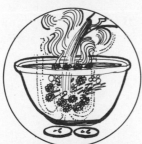

Take a large bowl, put a tablespoon of chamomile and 1 tablespoon of rosemary into it and pour boiling water on top of them. Lean over the bowl and cover your head with a large towel, making a tent over the bowl. The steam will open the pores, dislodge and loosen blackheads and bring spots to a head. Do not get too close to the water – about 12–24 in. (30–60 cm) is near enough. If the steam is too hot it can cause broken veins. After about 10 minutes wipe your face with skin tonic and you are ready for the face mask.

Apply your mayonnaise. (You won't need it all, so save some for your hair tomorrow.)

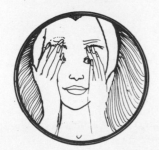

Lie down with eye pads on – use cucumber slices, wet tea bags or slices of raw potato.

Relax for 10–20 minutes, sleep if you can. Lie on your bed with your feet higher than your head, make sure that you are warm by covering yourself with a large blanket – and *relax*.

23

8.   Wash off the face mask with warm water and then apply a moisturizer.

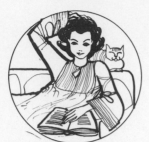

7.00   *Fruit-juice cocktail.* Try one of the delicious drinks on page 57 – the cucumber and mint juice which has a slightly diuretic effect, the Orange Sour which is incredibly refreshing, or have another glass of grape juice. Drink these juices out of your favourite glass, which somehow makes it more interesting and enjoyable.

7.30   Have a relaxing evening, read a book or magazine, or listen to some music.

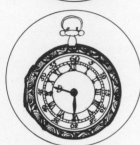

9.30   Go to bed early and dream about the fit, healthy and beautiful person you are going to be.

Day two

8.00   On waking go and get yourself a large glass of cold mineral water. Take it back to bed with you and relax, read or doze.

9.00   When you have woken up properly, stretch thoroughly in bed. Push back the covers and imagine you're being stretched on the rack, that your feet and hands are being pulled to touch the foot and head of your bed.
     Do the same bed exercises you did on Day One.

     Drink the juice of half a lemon in hot sugarless water.

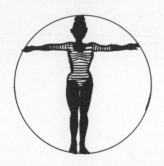

9.30   Spend at least thirty minutes exercising; concentrate on your problem areas (outlined in your mirror test). But, please; never miss out the warming-up exercises which you should do every day to loosen up, relieve tension, and generally keep you in basic trim (see *Exercises* section). You may be feeling slightly stiff after yesterday's attempts. Don't be half-hearted and give up. The more exercise you do the quicker the stiffness will wear off. Do them to music and finish off with five minutes of relaxation exercises.
     Take a quick, cool shower or bath, then dress comfortably.

10.15   *Tea.* Either lemon tea or a herb tea. This two-day blitz is a great time to experiment with teas. My favourite at the moment is one I bought in Ibiza, and appears to be a mixture of everything: anise, peppermint, rose petals, lavender, lemon balm and chamomile. Try various different combinations, some are really delicious (see page 31).

10.30   **Your posture**
     Are you round-shouldered or sway-backed? Do you get backache? Does your tummy stick out or your head stick forward?

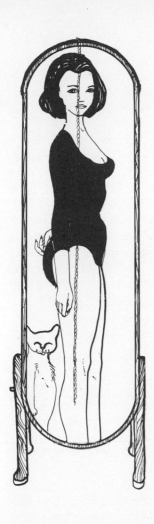

One of the first things that you notice about anyone is their carriage – how they hold themselves. If you stand and walk well you can disguise a multitude of faults. If you are over-weight it will conceal the fact, if you are short you will look tall. In fact, however you look, you will appear more attractive, slimmer and more confident if you walk tall.

Every muscle in your body should be working and keeping your body perfectly toned and upright in a straight line. Check your posture with this simple test. Hang a piece of string from the centre top of a full length mirror.

Stand sideways in front of it and look at yourself. Does the string bisect you in neat halves? Or do you bulge out drama-tically on either one or both sides of the string? Really study your posture. It is easier to do this with a friend because then you can criticize each other, rather than twisting your head to look in the mirror. If your body is in anything less than a perfectly straight line you need to start doing these exercises to re-train your slack muscles.

Pull in your bottom, tuck it right in and under. That will straighten your spine. Pull in your stomach, pull back your shoulders and hold up your head. Now look in the mirror and you will see how much better you look. Be conscious of your posture at all times, and do this simple exercise whenever you remember – frequently I hope.

A friend of mine who is an artist, and therefore crouched over a drawing board all day, has managed to maintain her posture by making herself a set of golden rules – The Four S's.

1. *String*. Imagine that a string is coming up from the middle of your head going up into the sky. It is as though you are a puppet, the string pulling the head upright and keeping your body in a straight line.
2. *Shoulders*. Remember to hold your shoulders back.
3. *Stomach*. Pull in your stomach.
4. *Smile*. She added this because one day she was walking along thinking of her 'S's' when she caught a glimpse of herself in a mirror – and she decided a smile was needed to counteract her grimaced look of concentration.

So just remember the four S's – string, shoulder, stomach and smile. Soon you will be walking like a king.

You should also try and train your children into the idea of good posture. My grandmother used to play a marvellous game with us. She would put books on our heads and we had to walk around the room balancing first one, then two, then three books. The classic way of training young children in deportment, and although old-fashioned, children usually enjoy these silly games, and it really does work. Start your children off in the right direction, in this way. Being taught good posture when they are young could save them a lifetime of backaches.

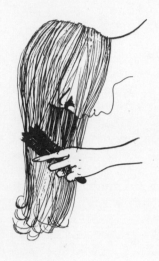

11.00 **Your hair**

Your scalp is just a continuation of the face and so it needs the same care – washing, massaging and creaming. If your hair is not as healthy or shiny as you would like it to be, take heart. As long as you are prepared to give it a little time and attention, it can easily be improved.

First check your diet. Are you eating correctly? For healthy hair you need lots of vitamin B, so check the nutrition section (page 36) and make sure to include foods rich in vitamin B in your diet. If your hair is in really bad condition then take extra brewers' yeast – about 6–8 tablets daily.

Now check your brushes and combs. Your brushes should preferably be bristle and your combs should have smooth edged teeth. Both should be kept spotlessly clean. You should brush your hair frequently to condition it and stimulate growth. Brush with your head hanging down, working up from the base of the scalp. Brushing like this increases the circulation, gives bounce to the hair – and exercises the bust muscles. Don't worry about all those hairs in your brush, a normal head loses, and replaces, about 50–100 hairs a day.

Conditioning. Use the remains of the mayonnaise you made yesterday to condition your hair. Make partings all over your head and apply your mayonnaise to the roots. Massage it well in with firm rotary movements all over your head, moving your scalp about and trying to loosen it. Apply any remaining mayonnaise to the rest of your hair. Wrap your head up in tin foil, and put a scarf or turban on top of that. If possible you want to leave this hair conditioner on for at least an hour (for 4 hours, if you're following my instructions!). (Practise doing turbans, they really are the most useful thing for anyone who is busy; the instant way to cover your dirty hair *and* make you look as though you just stepped out of a magazine – see page 76).

11.15 *Mid-morning snack.* It was at about this time that I began to feel the pangs of hunger and so I made up one of my favourite drinks, a mixture of yoghurt and tomato juice. It is relatively low in calories, delicious and *extremely* filling.

1 small carton yoghurt
(4–5 oz/100–125 g)
1 small can tomato juice
(4–5 oz/100–125 g)
Worcestershire sauce
Brewers' yeast (optional)

Mix the yoghurt (see page 55 for how to make your own) and tomato juice together, and add a few drops of Worcestershire sauce. If you are feeling like being really healthy add a teaspoon or two of brewers' yeast – I personally love the taste, but it is very distinctive and so only add a small amount at first.

11.30 Go for a long walk (or jog!) with your head still wrapped up in its tin-foil and scarf, or turban. This will make your head hot and the heat will make the conditioner work better.

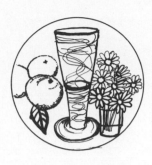

1.00 *Lunch.* A large bowl of vegetable juice, which is delicious, filling and very low in calories. Or have a bowl of hot or cold consommé. Then have a fresh, fruit juice – squeeze either one grapefruit or orange or mix the juices together. Sit back and enjoy it. Try sipping it through a straw to make it last longer.

1.30 Rest for half an hour with your feet higher than your head. Read one of those books or magazines you have always been meaning to read and never had the time to.

2.00 Have a really long luxurious bath. To have a bath in the middle of the day is wonderful – it is so marvellously pampering that it feels almost sinful!

Your bathroom ought to be your sanctuary. Having a bath can be a therapy in itself – the perfect way to soothe a tired body and restore one's peace of mind. The sheer luxury of letting the warm water envelop you and literally wash away any troubles and tiredness.

Elsewhere I will give you recipes for bath oils, bubble bath and bath salts. Learn to use them, and make your bath a haven of delight. Today use my favourite:

Milk and honey bath oil

2 eggs
¼ cup almond oil
¼ cup sunflower oil
2 tablespoons honey
2 teaspoons washing-up detergent
¼ cup vodka
½ cup milk
¼ teaspoon jasmin or sandalwood oil

Using the low speed on your electric beater (or use a hand beater) blend the eggs and oils together. Add the honey and detergent which act as emulsifiers and make it very thick. Then slowly, add in the vodka which gives the bath oil a dispersing quality and helps preserve the eggs and milk, and as this is only a small quantity there need be no fear that it will dry the skin. Continue beating and slowly add in the milk and then the perfumes, jasmin or sandalwood. Put a couple of tablespoons of this bath oil into your bath and you will be amazed to find that unlike most bath oils, it does not just rest on the surface but actually disperses into the water. This means that your skin will benefit from the oil throughout your bath – not only when you get in and out. Your skin will feel just like satin, all smooth, soft and silky. These quantities make enough bath oil for a couple of weeks, which, although the vodka is a preservative, should be used up within a month.

Lie back in your luxurious bath, listen to music and relax.

2.30 Have a small glass of fruit juice. Try some unsweetened apple juice because it is an aid to the digestion.

3.00 **Wash your hair**

You all know how to wash your hair, but do you do it correctly, and with as much care as it deserves?

1. First brush your hair (that prevents all those hairs clogging up the drain).

2. Wet your hair thoroughly.

3. Apply a little shampoo. I prefer to dilute it with water and beat it up so that I apply a lovely, light, frothy liquid.

4. Massage the shampoo into the hair, working with firm, rotary movements all over the scalp.

5. Rinse thoroughly. Carry on rinsing until your hair 'squeaks'. Hair that has not been properly rinsed might just have well not been washed at all. So rinse, and rinse, and rinse.

6. If you have very greasy hair you may wish to repeat the whole process and apply more shampoo, but for most people this is unnecessary – one thorough wash is enough.

7. The final rinse should be with cold water (or at least cool water) to tighten the pores.

8. Blot your hair dry with a towel. Don't brush or comb it until it is slightly dry, then set it.

If you wash your hair carefully like this, it can do absolutely no harm and so you can wash it as frequently as you wish.

4.00 **Body massage.** If you are lucky and are doing this with a friend, then do a complete massage which will take you about an hour. Otherwise massage yourself wherever you can reach – it's easy on the thighs, hips, tummy and even the upper arms. (See *Massage* section, pages 81–112.)

5.00 Have a cup of herb tea – why not try chamomile for its soothing qualities. Make a production out of having tea, using your favourite tea pot and best cups, and imagine that you are at a Japanese tea ceremony. Sit back and enjoy the luxury of having time to sip your tea.

5.30 **Give yourself a manicure**

Your hands and nails should have benefited from all the oil and cream you've been using for massage during the last two days. Now they need to be given the finishing touch – a professional manicure.

First gather all your equipment together. You will need: nail-varnish remover, emery boards, a bowl of warm soapy water and a nail brush, a towel, warm oil (or hand cream), cuticle cream, orange stick or hoof stick, buffer and nail varnishes, a base coat, colour and top coat. See pages 77–8 for easy recipes for hand and cuticle creams.

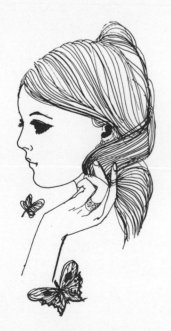

1. **Remove old nail varnish.** Wet a piece of cotton wool with remover, hold and press it against the whole nail for a second and then wipe off the varnish.

2. Shape your nails with an emery board, hold the emery board at a slant and sweep up, going in one direction only. Do not 'saw' as this will give you rough edges which causes nails to catch and tear.

3. Massage cuticle cream into the base of the nails, which

loosens and softens the cuticles and stimulates growth.

4. Gently push the cuticles back with a cotton-wool-wrapped orange stick – or better still a hoof stick. A hoof stick is rather like an orange stick with a rubber end. As I write I have just tried with the rubber tip of my pencil and this works almost as well. Gently ease back the cuticles, don't cut any hard skin as this seems to make the cuticle tougher. By giving yourself a proper complete manicure each week, you will find that the cuticles will gradually become softer.

5. Soak your hands in a bowl full of warm oil. Massage your hand working from the tips of the fingers right down to the wrists (see page 106). If you are too lazy to heat the oil, massage with your hand cream (page 77).

6. Soak your hands in warm soapy water and scrub the oil off the nails.

7. Dry the fingers and hands carefully, gently easing back the cuticles.

8. Buff your nails. This is optional but will greatly improve your nails whether you wear varnish or not. The buffing stimulates the circulation, encourages the growth and strengthens the nails. Buffing makes the nails look beautifully shiny, and I always think that plain naturally pearly nails look marvellous – but one has to work to achieve this natural look.

9. Apply base coat. You will find that it will go on easier after buffing.

10. Apply two or three coats of your nail varnish, allowing them to dry between applications. Professionals apply the varnish with only three strokes, one down each side and then one in the middle. Allow the nail varnish to dry and then apply a top coat to seal it all.

A complete manicure really is worth that little extra effort, as it only takes about half an hour and should last a week. Follow the advice a friend gave me and apply a fresh coat of either varnish or top coat every night, and you should never have chipped nail varnish again.

As you have everything gathered together, you could also give yourself a pedicure. Just follow the same procedure, but see also page 78.

6.30 *Fruit-juice cocktail.* Choose one of the drinks from the *Drink* section – or you could try prune juice, but it is a bit sweet and so only have a small glass. If you are feeling really adventurous you could try a glass of onion juice – it's a mild diuretic, but has a slightly strange taste!

7.00 More exercises if you can bear it. Do a few of your favourites.

7.30 Drink some cold mineral water.

By now you should be looking and feeling a thousand times better than you did two days ago. Every part of you should be glowing with health.

When I was writing and planning the *Two-day blitz* several clients and friends joined me in doing it. We all felt marvellous afterwards, even if a couple of us did cheat slightly. One friend simply couldn't resist eating an orange instead of having it as a juice and I'm afraid I couldn't resist a small glass of wine. But we all felt so much better that we kept up the good work by going on to do the *Seven-day campaign*.

8.00 Relax and congratulate yourself on keeping to your diet. But you had better go to bed early so that you don't sneak into the kitchen. Just before you go to bed have a cup of lime tea which is soothing and ensures a good sleep.

Herbs, flowers and leaves

Flowers and herbs have always been used in the search for health and beauty, and throughout this book you will continually be coming across references to them. They are needed for all the herbal teas in the *Two-day blitz*; you can add them to the bath and put them into the water when you steam your face; you can use infusions of the herbs in your cosmetics, your skin lotions, creams and masks.

To make an infusion pour a pint of boiling water over either two tablespoons of dried herbs, or a handful of fresh ones. Cover the jar or bowl tightly and let the herbs (or flowers) steep for about an hour. Strain and then use the infused water to wash with, or to add to any of the cosmetic recipes.

Different herbs have different properties. Here is a list of the ones I find the most useful, so that you can see their properties at a glance.

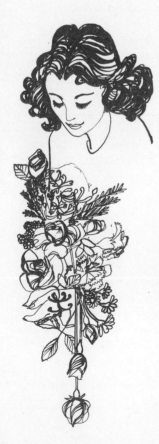

Basil – stimulating
Blackberry – healing and soothing
Calendular – soothing
Chamomile – soothing, bleaching, reduces puffiness
Comfrey – healing
Elderflower – softens and whitens the skin
Fennel – purifying, healing and said to delay wrinkles!
Lavender – stimulating, aromatic
Lemon peel – astringent, aromatic
Lime flowers – purifying and calming
Liquorice – stimulating
Marjoram – stimulating
Mint – purifying and stimulating
Nettles – increase the circulation and purifying
Orange peel – astringent and aromatic
Rosemary – stimulating, cleansing and said to clear the brain
Rose petals – soothing, healing and fragrant
Sage – antiseptic

Thyme – antiseptic
Yarrow – astringent.

As you can see the choice of herbs is endless. Use them either by themselves or make a mixture of your favourites and store those in a large flower jar ready for use. Add a couple of tablespoons to the water when you steam your face or put them (in a container of some type) into your bath.

Test for allergy
Herbs and flowers can, unfortunately – like everything else – cause allergic reactions. So you should always, therefore, treat them with respect. I was once terribly impressed by the healing qualities of the herb comfrey. It had cured some persistent sores on a friend's face and so I overdid it in experimenting on my *own* face. I came out in a hot prickly rash! (Comfrey is, of course, a marvellous herb, used in medieval times to heal fractures and was known as knitbone: it's a cell regenerative, containing allantoin – so don't please be put off it!)

If you think you might be allergic to something, give yourself a 'patch test'. Apply some of the herbal solution behind your ears and cover it with a sticking plaster. After an hour check for redness or swelling. If there is none, the chances are you can use that herb quite safely.

Herb teas
Herb teas are a marvellous addition to one's diet. I have noticed that when I recommend herb teas there is sometimes a resistance: people think it will be time-consuming to make the teas, or that their taste leaves something to be desired. It is true that some herb teas are slightly bitter but by mixing a couple together you can easily overcome that problem, and on the question of time, it is just as simple to make herb tea as it is any other tea. The method is the same, a pint of boiling water poured over 1–2 teaspoons of dried herbs.

There are masses of herb teas which really are absolutely delicious. And on this *Two-day blitz* you have ample time to experiment and find your favourites. You aren't supposed to be eating and so fill yourself up with herb teas instead. They all have different properties, some stimulating, some purifying and others soothing. They not only taste good, they also do you good!

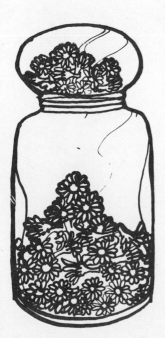

Anise tea
This gentle, delicate tasting tea has a marvellously calming effect on the stomach if you suffer from indigestion, wind, or a stomach ache of any kind. (Anise, carraway and fennel are all an aid to digestion.)

Chamomile tea
This is a soothing tea which calms the nerves and is thought to prevent nightmares. It has a slightly strange taste which people tend to either love or hate – try mixing it with other teas if you fall into the latter category. The herbalist Parkinson in 1640 had this to say about it:

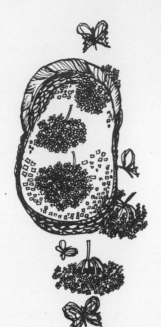

'Chamomile is put to divers and sundry uses, both for pleasure and profit, both for sick and sound, in bathing to comfort and strengthen the sound and to ease pains in the diseased.' It is also said to help earache and toothache.

Elderflower tea

This is simply delicious, and is considered an excellent blood purifier.

Fennel tea

Not only useful as an aid to digestion and for settling the stomach, fennel is also said to help make you slender. Its ancient Greek name was *Marathon* from '*maraino*', to grow thin, and one comes across frequent references to this virtue.

Chewing fennel seeds also helps to reduce the appetite.

Lime tea

Lime or linden tea (*Tilleul*) is drunk in tremendous quantities in Europe. It is calming and soothing. In many households you are given a cup of linden tea before retiring, to ensure a good night's rest.

Mint tea

1½ tablespoons green tea
Handful of fresh or dried whole mint leaves (the menthe virdis variety)
1 lump sugar, substitute with sweeteners to taste

In Morocco one is constantly handed little glasses of this deliciously refreshing and stimulating drink, the preparation of which is considered an art. There are many ways of making it. Here is one version adapted from Claudia Roden's marvellous book *Middle Eastern Cooking*. Heat the teapot. Add the tealeaves and pour a little boiling water over them. Swirl around and quickly pour the water out again, taking care not to lose the leaves. Add mint and sugar (sweetener) to taste and pour in 1½–2 pints (about 1 litre) boiling water. Allow to infuse for 5–8 minutes. Serve in little glasses.

According to Culpeper, mint 'stirs up venery, or bodily lust' – so beware!

Mixed teas

(i) 4 teaspoons mint
3 teaspoons liquorice (break a stick up into small pieces)
2 teaspoons chamomile
2 teaspoons lavender
1 teaspoon sage
1 teaspoon anise

(ii) 1 teaspoon parsley
1 teaspoon fennel
1 teaspoon elderflowers
½ teaspoon carraway

(iii) 2 teaspoons mint
2 teaspoons sage
1 teaspoon rosemary

By mixing the different herbs one can make teas which taste interestingly exotic.

When I was in Ibiza, the old woman in the herbalist gave me a tea which seems to contain practically everything, a marvellous mixture of different flowers and herbs. Since then I have taken to mixing my own and here are a few suggestions.

In each of these recipes mix all the herbs together and store them in an airtight container. To make the tea mix a couple of teaspoons to a pint of boiling water. Allow to stand for a minute and then drink and enjoy it. If you have a sweet tooth sweeten either with honey or sweeteners.

These teas all have the most calming effect – so if you have been feeling irritable have a cup of delicious, aromatic tea to soothe your aggravated nerves.

Diet & Dieting

Before going on a diet you really ought to check with your doctor that it is safe for you to do so. Most normally healthy people don't bother, but you must go immediately if you feel at all unwell or peculiar.

We are going to turn your home into a health farm and began your new healthy life by going on the *Two-day blitz*, living on liquids only. This will lead into the *Seven-day campaign*, which is a strict diet, and from that we will progress to the *Three-week health kick*.

I think that it will make your dieting more interesting if you know something about nutrition. After all, you are supposed to be at a health farm, so you should know something about what food is healthy and why!

Diet and nutrition

We all know that there are three basic nutrients in food – proteins, carbohydrates and fats.

We need food not only to provide us with energy, but also to supply the body with hundreds of different chemical compounds which are necessary for good health. Hardly any food contains only one nutrient; most are a combination of water, carbohydrate, fat and protein with vitamins and minerals in smaller quantities.

When planning the diets I have been extremely careful to include all the nutrients that you need to keep you healthy.

Proteins

The word protein means 'of first importance'. They are essential for the growth and repair of the body – any excess is converted into glucose and used to provide energy. Proteins contain amino acids, which are vital for the body. These amino acids are divided into two groups – essential and non-essential. The essential amino acids, of which there are eight, cannot be made in the body and so have to be supplied by your food, whereas the non-essential amino acids can be made from any excess of other amino acids in the diet. Proteins containing all the essential amino acids are known as 'complete' proteins and most animal proteins fall into this category. Vegetables and nuts tend to be incomplete proteins, but if they are eaten together, mixing the varieties, they complement each other and increase their value. Amino acids cannot be stored and are most efficiently used if an assortment is provided each time you eat – for example bread and cheese, meat and vegetables, and fish and chips.

Foods high in protein include liver, meat, poultry, bacon, ham; white fish and oily fish; eggs, milk, cheese; soya beans, wheatgerm,

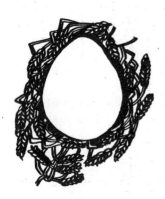

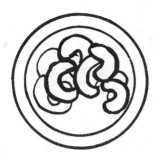

brewers' yeast; almonds, cashew nuts, peanuts, lentils, dried beans and sunflower seeds (which contain nearly as much as steak).

I have included most of these foods in the diets. It is always advisable to eat something from this list every day, not only for your general health but also for your looks. Without protein the skin becomes dry, scaly and sallow.

Fats

Fats provide heat and energy in a more concentrated way than carbohydrates. Fat is digested relatively slowly, and by staying longer in the stomach prevents hunger pangs – extremely useful on a diet. Fats tend to be high in calories and so if you are calorie-counting you should restrict their intake. When carbohydrate-counting this restriction is not necessary.

Animal fats usually contain small amounts of vitamins A and D, and cholesterol, while vegetable fats contain carotene (which is converted by the body into vitamin A) and vitamin E, but no cholesterol.

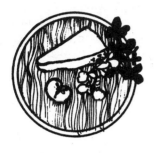

Foods rich in fat are butter, margarine, oils, meat, milk, cheese, nuts and fatty fish (herrings, mackerel, tuna and sardines).

Carbohydrates

Carbohydrates, our main source of heat and energy, are divided into three major groups: sugar, starch and cellulose. Although all carbohydrates absorbed by the body provide the same amount of energy they have different effects. Sugar, for instance, has *no* nutritional value at all – in other words it can be termed an 'empty calorie'. Until recently, sugar was only eaten in small quantities, obtained from natural foods such as milk, honey and fruit, but now sucrose (our refined sugar is made from sucrose) is used liberally in sweets, jams, cakes and biscuits. This not only provides us with an alarming number of calories but can also cause tooth decay, indigestion and obesity.

Starch forms the bulk of energy of most plants and the bulk of man's food energy. Some starches, such as wheatgerm, flour, oatmeal, lentils and bread, contain the B vitamins and so some should be included in our diet.

Cellulose, also known as fibre, or roughage, is an essential part of diet because it assists in the passage of waste materials through the intestines. When you are slimming it bulks out your diet and so makes you feel full. Cellulose is the fibrous structure in vegetables, and is found, for example, in the skin of apples or potatoes, or in the string in celery. Bran is a rich source of cellulose, which is why it's so lauded as an aid to the bowels.

Foods high in carbohydrates: bread, oatmeal, potatoes, flour, lentils, pasta and beans.

Foods high in sugar – which should be avoided: syrup, jam, biscuits, cakes, tinned fruit, chocolates, ice cream, dried fruit, soft drinks and spirits.

Vitamins

Until vitamins were discovered in 1915 it was thought that proteins, fats and carbohydrates were the only ingredients necessary for a balanced diet. Vitamins are organic compounds found in a variety of foods, and minute quantities of them are essential to good health.

Insufficient vitamins in your diet leads to stunted growth and a general feeling of malaise. But the theory that as we need vitamins and they do us good, then large quantities would do us *more* good, is not necessarily true. Vitamins are one of two types: water-soluble (B and C) and fat-soluble (A, D, E and K). Water-soluble vitamins are usually measured in milligrams (mgs), fat soluble vitamins in international units (I.U.'s). Taking excessive amounts of water-soluble vitamins is perfectly safe as they are simply eliminated, but if you take very large doses of the fat soluble vitamins they are stored in the body and can cause ill effects.

'*To go beyond is as wrong as to fall short.*'
Confucius, 6th century B.C.

A tremendous number of people supplement their diets with vitamin tablets, and these are useful if you are deficient in a particular vitamin or are not eating a nutritionally sound diet. But vitamin therapy is a new science and new discoveries are being made all the time. In nature, vitamins come in combinations – one compound will help another to be utilized efficiently by the body, and indiscriminate use of pills can upset this balance. If possible it is much better to take all the vitamins you need by eating properly and not by 'pill-popping'. Eat the food – not the pills.

Vitamin A
Vitamin A helps maintain smooth, soft, healthy skin. It aids growth and repair of the surface tissues and mucous membranes. It helps vision in dim light – a deficiency results in night blindness and general weakness of the eyes – as well as skin problems.

Vitamin A is fat-soluble and so excessive quantities can be poisonous – this excess would usually be obtained from massive doses of pills or living almost exclusively on vitamin A, as in the case of the man who drank eight pints of carrot juice daily.

A friend who suffered from goose flesh on her upper arms found that when she took 5,000 I.U.'s of vitamin A daily for about a week the roughness disappeared. Do try it if you have 'goose-fleshy', red patchy skin or even warts. I have also found that if people suffer from excessively rough, dry skin and they take either cod-liver oil or halibut-liver oil capsules, the improvement in their skin is miraculous. If vitamin A is applied externally to the skin it can help to clear up acne, sores and wounds.

The most concentrated form of vitamin A comes from fish-liver oils – halibut or cod. Liver and kidneys are another rich source followed by dairy products, eggs and margarine. Vegetables also supply vitamin A to our diet, in particular carrots and green vegetables, and the darker the green the higher the vitamin content.

The recommended daily dietary allowance of vitamin A, according to the Manual of Nutrition issued by the Ministry of Agriculture, Fisheries and Food, is 750 mgs. This is roughly the equivalent of ½ oz/15 g liver, 2½ oz/65 g butter or margarine, 1½ medium-sized carrots, 2½ oz/65 g spinach or 4 oz/100 g cheddar cheese.

Vitamin B complex

The B vitamins are essential for maintaining healthy nerves and have been called the anti-stress vitamins. They are active in the production of energy from carbohydrates and in the metabolism of fats and proteins. The health of your hair and skin also depends on an adequate intake.

The B vitamins function together and are found in the same foods. The most commonly known B complex vitamins are Thiamin (B_1), Riboflavin (B_2) and Niacin (B_3).

A lack of the B vitamins causes depression, tiredness, irritability, nervousness and insomnia. It can also give rise to anaemia, a poor appetite and indigestion. Acne, grey and falling hair, cracks around the mouth and sensitive eyes can also all be indications of a lack of vitamin B.

A vitamin B deficiency can be fairly common in people who drink and smoke to excess, or who eat too much sugar. Stress and the taking of antibiotics, also deplete the body's supply. In all these circumstances it is advisable to eat more food containing vitamin B (or take a vitamin B complex tablet regularly).

The B vitamins are water-soluble and any excess taken is excreted; it is therefore important to replace them each day.

If your hair is listless, breaking and generally in bad condition, a marked improvement can be achieved by taking vitamin B (in hairdressing salons they recommend 6–8 tablets of brewers' yeast but a tablespoon of the powder is stronger and so try that first – I know that it is an acquired taste but surely it is worth acquiring for the sake of shiny, healthy hair). Vitamin B also does wonders for your skin (anyone suffering from acne should take large quantities) and it is said to be a natural anti-wrinkle aid – I knew I was eating all that brewers' yeast and liver for something!

Brewers' yeast is the richest source of the B vitamins, followed by whole grain cereals, wheatgerm and milk. It is also found in smaller quantities in vegetables, fruit, nuts and liver.

Vitamin C (ascorbic acid)

Vitamin C is essential for producing strong connective tissue. It maintains the collagen fibres in the skin, ligaments and bones. For this reason it is important in the treating of wounds and burns because it speeds up the healing process. If you are having surgery, large doses of vitamin C help in a rapid recovery, and in some hospitals in America large doses are given to patients who have been badly burned.

Vitamin C reduces the effects of some allergy-producing substances and fights bacterial infections and fevers. For this reason it is often used in treating colds. Although the scientific evidence is still contested, I am sure that large doses of vitamin C do help to prevent colds; if you feel a cold coming take some vitamin C every hour – either eat an orange or take a vitamin C tablet. I find that this usually prevents the cold or at least gets rid of it very quickly.

I have also been told that if you give vitamin C every hour to children who are suffering from infections and fevers, it will bring down their

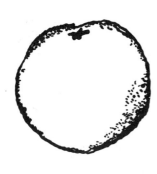

temperatures and hasten their recovery.

It is thought that smoking greatly reduces the body's ability to absorb vitamin C, which is also impaired by high fever, antibiotics and pain killers. Under stress you use up vitamin C very rapidly and so for all these conditions increase your vitamin C intake.

Vitamin C is water-soluble and cannot be stored in the body. In fact most vitamin C is eliminated about 3–4 hours after taking it. For this reason, and because the body can only absorb a certain amount at a time, it is better to take several small doses of vitamins in a day rather than one massive dose.

'Time and care spent on health is an investment in yourself.'
Mae West

The recommended intake is about 50–80 mgs daily – that is the equivalent of about two oranges or a glass of fresh orange juice. Dr Linus Pauling, however, says the optimum daily intake should be from 1,000–9,000 mgs.

The need for vitamin C increases with age because of the need to regenerate the collagen.

Vitamin C is readily lost in storage and cooking. The main source of vitamin C is citrus fruits. The pith and white segments of the citrus fruit contain riboflavonoids, a substance which helps the vitamin C to be absorbed and work more effectively. Green vegetables, rose hips, blackcurrants and potatoes also contain vitamin C.

Vitamin D

Vitamin D is sometimes known as the 'sunshine' vitamin. Most of our vitamin D is obtained by the reaction of the ultra-violet rays with a substance (Ergosterol) in the skin converting it into vitamin D. It is also available from a few foods, the main source being fish-liver oils, fatty fish, eggs, butter and fortified margarine. Vitamin D is best utilized when taken with vitamin A: that is the reason that fish-liver oils (rich in both vitamin A and D) are such a good source. Vitamin D is essential to the absorption of calcium and phosphorus. A deficiency results in deformed bones, poor teeth, rickets and nervous irritability.

During pregnancy, lactation and the menopause, the need for vitamin D increases. The Ministry of Agriculture, Fisheries and Food recommends 2·5 mg daily. To get the equivalent of this you would need to eat, for example, 1 oz/25 g sardines or 1 oz/25 g fortified margarine. An adequate supply of calcium and phosphorus are essential if vitamin D is to be utilized efficiently by the body.

Some research in America has shown that taking vitamins A and D can reduce the frequency and severity of colds. During one winter in Norway I noticed that the Norwegians took a cod-liver oil tablet each day, which, on the evidence of this research, seems an extremely sensible thing to do.

Vitamin E

Although the many claims for the miraculous effects of vitamin E have yet to be proved, they are extremely interesting. Vitamin E is an anti-oxidant, that is, it opposes the oxidation of substances in the body, and as the ageing of the cells is caused by oxidation, vitamin E is thought to be useful in retarding the ageing process. Oils and fats containing vitamin E are less likely to go rancid. Vitamin E promotes healing both internally and externally. It prevents or dissolves scar tissue and can aid in the healing of burns and abrasions. I have also found that it helps to remove old acne scars, and that dry, itchy skin, which sometimes occurs with age, can also be relieved by the application of vitamin E. When using vitamin E externally it is a good idea to take it orally as well, as the two methods complement each other.

Vitamin E is thought to be connected with fertility and reproduction, and it has been found to be helpful in regulating the menstrual rhythm and alleviating menstrual pain. It has also been used with success on the treatment of hot flushes and headaches during menopause.

A deficiency in vitamin E could result in the premature ageing of the skin, shrinkage of collagen and connective tissue. Vitamin E and C work together to keep the blood vessels flexible and healthy. It is thought that the brown spots that sometimes occur with age on the hands maybe due to a lack of vitamin E.

When iron and vitamin E are taken simultaneously the absorption of each is impaired. They should be taken separately, preferably with as much as an eight-hour interval.

The National Research Council in America recommends a daily dose of about 12 I.U.'s for adults, which should be increased to 15 I.U.'s during pregnancy and lactation. However, in her book *Let's Eat Right* Adelle Davies, the famous nutritionalist, puts the dosage as high as 100 I.U.'s daily.

Vitamin E is fat-soluble, but excessive doses of vitamin E are excreted and all effects of vitamin E disappear after three days. If mineral oil is taken as a laxative it depletes the body of vitamin E.

Most food contains some vitamin E but the main sources are wheatgerm, brown bread, vegetable oils, nuts, grains and eggs.

Vitamin F (unsaturated fatty acids)
Vitamin F makes it easier for oxygen to be taken by the blood stream to all tissues, organs and cells.

A lack of vitamin F can cause dry skin, eczema, dandruff, lifeless hair and allergic conditions.

The National Research Council in America recommends that at least 1% of one's total calories are from unsaturated fatty acids. Eating a great deal of carbohydrates and saturated fats, such as butter and cream, increases the need for vitamin F. It is a fat-soluble vitamin. The main sources are lecithin, wheatgerm, and vegetable oils such as soy oil, sunflower oil and corn oil.

Minerals
To benefit from vitamins it is necessary to have a balanced intake of minerals.

Approximately 5% of the body's weight is made up of minerals. They are needed by the body for normal growth and repair of tissues, muscles and bones. They help to control the fluid in the body, are constituents of bones and teeth, and they are necessary for the release and utilization of energy.

There are seven major minerals which are known to be vital to health. These are calcium, iron, phosphorus, magnesium, sodium, chlorine and potassium. The remainder are also essential but are needed in much smaller quantities. These are known as trace elements. They include iodine, fluorine, cobalt, chronium, copper, magnesium and zinc.

Foods rich in minerals: molasses, honey and seaweed.

Calcium

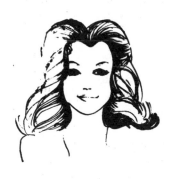

Calcium is the most abundant mineral in the body, essential in the formation and maintenance of bones and teeth. It assists in muscle action, normal clotting of the blood and nerve function. The nutritionalist, Adelle Davies, called calcium a natural tranquillizer and recommends its use against a number of complaints. If you suffer from insomnia take 2–3 calcium tablets with a warm milky drink just before going to bed – and if the insomnia persists take a calcium tablet with milk every hour.

It has also been recommended that women who suffer from premenstrual tension, back-ache and cramps, should take calcium every hour until they are gone. Again a number of us tried this and thought that it definitely helped; it seemed to dispel fatigue, irritability and pain. One friend even thought that it cured her migraine, so it is well worth a try. Relax yourself by taking a couple of calcium pills before going to the dentist. An increase of calcium may be needed for young children; during pregnancy and lactation; and with the onset of the menopause. For adults the recommended dietary allowance is between 800–1,400 mg – the equivalent of about $\frac{1}{2}$ pint/300 ml of milk. (Milk contains about 120 mg per 100 gms.)

The main sources of calcium are milk, yoghurt and cheese and it is for this reason that they should be included in your diet.

Iron

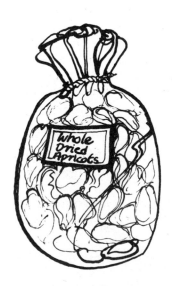

Iron helps in protein metabolism and is necessary for haemoglobin (the red pigment in blood) formation, and the transportation of oxygen to the muscles and tissues.

A deficiency can give rise to anaemia, weakness, pale skin and constipation.

During pregnancy and menstruation more iron may be needed by the body and so eat lots of iron-rich food.

The main sources of iron are liver, offal and dried apricots. In order to increase the absorption of iron, vitamin C should be eaten at the same time (in our diet I have always taken this into account).

Phosphorus

Phosphorus works with calcium to build bones and teeth. It also helps to liberate and utilize the energy from food.

It is present in nearly all food and a deficiency is highly unlikely. Rich sources are yeast extract, cheddar cheese, peanuts, chicken, meat and fish.

Magnesium

Magnesium is needed for the functioning of some enzymes and to enable the body to utilize food energy. A deficiency is again unlikely as it is present in most food, especially peanuts, yeast, and soy beans.

Sodium and chlorine

Sodium and chlorine maintain the body's water balance and are essential for muscle and nerve activity.

Sodium chloride (salt) is contained in all the body fluids. Under normal circumstances we get all the salt we need in our food – about 4 gms per day – and in fact most people take in as much as 5–20 gm a day by adding extra salt to their food. Consequently a deficiency only arises if there is excessive water loss from sweating – after strenuous exercise, for instance, or in a very hot climate – in which case extra salt should be taken to prevent muscle cramps.

Potassium

Potassium has a complementary action with sodium in the working of the cells and muscle, nerve and kidney activity.

Potassium is found in most food, the main sources being yeast extract, fresh fruit and vegetables (especially radishes, tomatoes and bananas) egg yolk and yoghurt. But if the vegetables are soaked or boiled and the water discarded, most of the potassium is thrown away.

If you take diuretics or purgatives you eliminate potassium and that can cause a deficiency.

I have read that a deficiency in potassium can lead to water retention, and as this is such a common problem with women, I think it is wise to follow the country tradition of drinking all the water that our vegetables are cooked in – even if it doesn't diminish the water retention, it is so loaded with other vitamins and minerals that it can only do us good.

'Use three physicians still
First Doctor Quiet,
Next Doctor Merry Man
And Doctor Dyet.'
From *Schola Salernitana,* transl. by Sir James Harrington, 1607

Trace minerals

Iodine regulates the metabolism and production of energy and is needed by the thyroid glands. The most reliable source of iodine is sea food. Kelp is an extremely rich source; it is a good idea to use iodized salt.

Fluorine is thought to reduce tooth decay. Drinking water is the most important source but it is also available in tea and sea food.

Cobalt works as part of the vitamin E complex – a lack of it causes anaemia.

Chromium is essential for the utilization of sugar (glucose).

Copper is associated with the work of enzymes.

Magnesium again acts as an enzyme activator and in the maintenance of the sex-hormone production. Found in wheatgerm, nuts, bran and green, leafy vegetables.

Zinc aids in metabolism and helps the healing process. It is present in a wide variety of food, especially green leafy vegetables.

Diet supplements

When reading about nutrition certain foods keep cropping up as being highly nutritious. These unusual foods, which are often delicious, could make an interesting supplement to your diet.

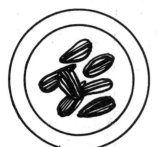

Sunflower seeds

The protein content of sunflower seeds is nearly as high as that of steak – they contain more protein than all other seeds. They are rich in vitamins B, D and E and minerals. About 2 oz/59 g (that's about half a cup) contain 280 calories and 10 carbohydrates. They are absolutely delicious and I eat them instead of sweets or whenever I'm starving and in need of a quick snack, to raise energy and stave off hunger.

Seaweed

Seaweed is full of iodine, needed by the thyroid gland which controls our metabolism. The theory is that by taking seaweed (kelp) it may increase the speed with which we burn up fat, thus helping us to lose weight. Whether that is true or not, seaweed is a tremendously rich source of minerals, vitamins and protein. It has been claimed that taking seaweed can prevent colds, help relieve arthritis and generally improve cell regeneration and fingernails.

In Hong Kong seaweed (*nori*) is taken as a snack and given to children to keep their hair black. It tastes delicious, slightly salty and crunchy. In Ireland I was once given *dulse* to eat and the girl in the shop told me that she had dulse sandwiches for lunch every day. Since reading about the miraculous effects of seawood, I have tried to add it to my diet in the form of kelp tablets, or better still kelp powder. It is really quite nice if you add it to yoghurt or tomato juice, stews or soups, or use it for cooking instead of salt.

Lecithin

Lecithin is found in every cell of the body. It is an excellent source of two of the B vitamins and essential fatty acids and is also an emulsifier which is thought to help in our metabolism, in the breaking down and redistribution of fat and cholesterol. Lecithin is rich in phosphorus and there is an old German saying 'No phosphorus, no brain!' Lecithin is found in the soya bean, egg yolks and polyunsaturated oils. The granules are tasteless and so can easily be added to our Health Cereal (page 63).

Liquorice

Liquorice is a laxative with diuretic properties which was once used to combat cramps caused by stomach ulcers and to quench the thirst when going into battle. I have read that Napoleon (who suffered from stomach aches) habitually chewed the liquorice root which eventually blackened his teeth.

Sesame seeds

These contain vitamin T which helps in correcting anaemia and in re-establishing blood coagulation. I was also told that they help a fading memory. (Since then I've hopefully been adding a couple of teaspoons to my Health Cereal each day – I don't think that my memory has improved but they taste delicious!)

Desiccated liver tablets

Ideally you should eat liver at least once a week. All the books on nutrition point out how good it is for us but this is another food with an acquired taste. You'll either love it or hate it. If you fall into the latter category you should take desiccated liver tablets which contain most of the original nutrients. As I said before, if you do eat liver, remember to have it at the same time as some citrus fruit, as the vitamin C helps the absorption of the iron.

Brewers' yeast

I have already gone into the marvels of brewers' yeast. (See vitamin B, page 36). This is one of the foods which features in every single book on nutrition, because it is one of the best sources of vitamin B.

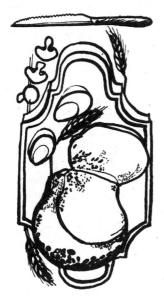

Wheatgerm

You will have noticed that this keeps cropping up in the lists of minerals and vitamins. It is well worth getting into the habit of eating this delicious cereal.

All things in moderation

There are numerous conflicting reports of what constitutes a healthy, balanced diet. Everyone has a pet theory, books and magazines all extol their personal bias. Even the same report, or experiment, can be covered very differently by the Press. For instance, in 1971, discussing the question of harmful mercury levels in food, the *Guardian* said, 'Fish mercury levels too high', whereas *The Times* on the same day wrote, 'Mercury, no danger levels in food'. Both were quoting the same report issued by the Ministry of Agriculture.

People even misunderstand the most common of foods – bread. The controversy over white versus brown bread has been raging for years, and really there is no satisfactory answer. It depends on what is needed by the body at any given time. As Allan Cameron said in his book, *Food, Facts and Fallacies*, wholemeal bread contains more fibre, and it could be said that it is better for health as this has a laxative effect. But the extra roughage also means that smaller amounts of nutrients are absorbed by the body so that one could conclude that white bread, with its added vitamins and nutrients, is healthier than wholemeal. In other words, both are good for you and it really depends on what is needed at any time by your body and which you prefer.

There is also the mistaken illusion that everything natural is good for you. But most of the really powerful poisons are natural, among them conium of hemlock (that killed Socrates) and the hallucinogenic L.S.D. of the ergot fungus. Nutmeg can give euphoria and produce addiction. And potatoes and spinach, whether sprayed with insecticide or not, contain certain toxic elements. Hens' eggs, whether free range or battery, contain a natural carcinogenic substance. And even salt, one of the oldest of preservatives, can make you ill if taken in excess.

Almost anything taken in excess can be harmful. There was the alarming case of the health-food addict who drank himself to death on carrot juice. His wife said that no one prescribed it – he just thought it was the right way to eat. Apart from all the carrot juice (which is vitamin A) he also took vitamin A tablets. At the inquest a doctor said that the vitamin A poisoning produced a condition indistinguishable from alcoholic poisoning. He was killed by the 8 pints of carrot juice he drank daily.

Even the belief that animal fats contribute to coronary heart disease and high cholesterol levels, which was widely believed a while ago, is now under review. In experiments done recently there appears to be no link between diet and the levels of cholesterol and fat in the blood. And even after all the 'anti-fat' propaganda, when surveys were done, no change in the number of heart attacks were found. So although high levels of cholesterol in the blood are associated with heart disease medical researchers are again looking for the unknown factor which causes it. In a recent report in the *New Scientist*, a doctor suggested that the best preventative measure is exercise: 'It's fitness, not fatness that counts.' This whole area still seems controversial.

'Because sugar is not arsenic, many graves are full.'
Proverb

One thing that everyone seems to be in agreement about is that we eat far too much sugar. In his book on sugar, *Pure, White and Deadly*, the famous nutritionist, Professor J. Yudkin, tells us that in the past 200 years our consumption of sugar has risen so dramatically that in two weeks people now eat the same amount that used to be consumed in a year. We find ourselves eating sugar without even realizing it. A tremendous amount of prepacked food has large quantities added; soups, tinned food, soft drinks, cereals, and of course biscuits and sweets. Start reading the labels and you will be amazed to find it in the most unlikely foods. All this sugar that we consume – on average in the U.K. about 5 oz/125 g per person a day – has no nutritional value. Its only contribution to our diet is to give us extra calories and probably to make us fat. Sugar is what is known as an empty calorie and if a large proportion of our total calorie intake each day consists of sugar, it is quite likely that we may be lacking some of the nutrients we would get from other, more valuable, food.

So remember, sugar is useless to you and whether you are trying to become slim, or just remain healthy, I suggest you should eat as little of it as possible. A Saudi Arabian doctor told me that in his country people eat dates and honey cakes and baklava every morning, but that they don't eat anything else sweet for the rest of the day. We in Europe, on the other hand, eat less sugar at one time, but we spread our consumption through the day. We have sugar with everything – our tea, coffee, biscuits, puddings and drinks.

His theory was that when you eat all the sugar in one sitting as with the dates and baklava, the sugar is not metabolized properly and gets eliminated. But if you split up the eating of sugar, it is stored in the body in the form of fat.

The time of day when you eat your food is important. Food eaten at night tends to turn to fat – because we don't work it off. By the same token we ought to eat the bulk of our calories in the morning. We should eat a really substantial breakfast, a token lunch and a light supper. I'd like to see a study on fat and thin people and the correlation between their weight and the time they took the bulk of their food. In the meantime you might care to do your own research – vary the times of your main meal and see if that reduces your weight.

But the general conclusion I have come to is that a little of everything does you good. I know – isn't it boring – one is always longing for a magic formula which will have us bursting with energy, healthy and slim. But it seems to me that there are no magic formulas, no short cuts to either health or slimness – just good plain nutritional food. *In other words all things in moderation.*

Why are we overweight?

'*Better too fat than too thin.*'
Woody Allen

Primarily because we eat too much. There are many causes of over-eating, but one of the simplest is that we fall prey to persuasion from advertising or from food arrayed temptingly in shops and super-markets. It is very easy to over-indulge and then find that one has gained weight, especially as so many packaged, frozen or tinned pro-ducts contain added sugar and starch, thus accustoming us to a fairly high intake of sweet food. Of course there are many different reasons for eating more food than is strictly necessary. If you are ner-vous or tense, anxious or unhappy, you often eat a lot as a kind of compensation. Conversely happy people might not care about their figures and thus also become too fat.

It sounds easier than it is to cut down the amount one eats. Doctors and dieticians now realize that they have to tackle the *causes* of over-eating as much as prescribing diets. There are many books and maga-zine articles reflecting this new angle of research which suggest ways of analysing the reasons for overeating.

Many people try and convince themselves that their excess weight is due to glandular trouble, water retention or heavy bones and muscles. But this is highly unlikely and very rarely the case.

Here are some of the many – and I'm afraid, patently thin – reasons given for cheating on a diet:

I am really on a diet, but I will eat this because . . .
1. Everyone likes me the way I am – plump.
2. No one ever notices anyway.
3. I'll start properly again on Monday.
4. I've hardly eaten a thing today.
5. I've eaten so much I might as well give up.
6. In this cold weather I need more food.
7. In this hot weather the pounds will 'melt' off anyway.
8. This restaurant is so good, to hell with my diet.
9. It would be rude to my hostess after she has cooked such a delicious meal.

10. There is only spaghetti on the menu and I can't sit here and eat nothing.
11. When I am cooking I have to taste.
12. At my height it doesn't show.
13. I've worked so hard today I need a bit more energy.
14. I've given up smoking and need pampering.
15. It seems a waste to throw away this little leftover.
16. I missed breakfast and need something now – even if it is a sticky bun.
17. I am greedy, self-indulgent and weak-willed.

Does any of that seem familiar to you? I'm sure it does, because it's hard to find anyone who has *not* been on some sort of diet over the last year or so – we seem almost obsessional about being thin.

Golden rules

But if you want to diet, either in a 'crash' fashion (see page 53) or more slowly and sensibly, coupling your desire for thinness with a desire for health, here are some golden rules to start you off along the way:

1. BEFORE YOU DIET RECORD YOUR INTAKE

There are hundreds of tricks to dieting, and the first is to find out exactly what you are eating now and why it is making you fat.

People frequently tell me that they simply can't understand it, 'they don't eat anything', and yet they are still fat. Something, or someone, is wrong. The first thing you have to do, before you even begin to diet, is to record everything you eat and when you eat it. Write down absolutely *everything* and when and where you ate it. You will be quite horrified at the quantity you've eaten and if you calculate the calorie total it will give you a nasty shock. One way of doing this, although expensive (but worth it in the end), is every time you eat anything, put the equivalent amount in a large saucepan. At the end of the day you will be able to see just how much you have piled into your stomach. A horrifying thought!

2. FIND OUT WHEN YOU ARE HUNGRY

Take particular notice of the times when you eat but are unaware of doing it. For instance all that tasting whilst cooking, the 'tidying up' of children's tea, or finishing off those bits in the fridge. By knowing and recognizing the times of day that you feel hungry you can make sure to have some sensible food then. When dieting never allow yourself to feel so hungry and desperate that your will-power evaporates and you will eat any or everything.

3. WHAT CAN'T YOU LIVE WITHOUT?

Most of us have a weakness for some food or other. If you hate meat or eggs the high protein diet is obviously not the one for you. You must be realistic and face up to your weaknesses. For instance I love wine and cheddar cheese, and a diet of more than a week without these two items is extremely difficult for me to bear. Of course you could do totally without but why punish yourself? It is much more sensible to admit to your weaknesses and incorporate them into your diet. I have one client who simply loves chocolates and so she counts calories carefully and in this way can allow herself an occasional sweet even when she's on the strictest of diets.

This realistic approach will mean that you have much more chance of sticking to your diet. Remember it is the long-term effect we're after – a healthy diet for life.

4. BOREDOM FACTOR

'Keep on plodding, and you won't go backwards.' Sally Mallam

All dieting, however varied, becomes boring. You want to rebel against your self-imposed regime. When this happens and I'm afraid it always does, you must do something about it quickly! Go to the cinema or play tennis. Try on clothes both to see how much better they look now, and to remind yourself, perhaps, that there is still a way to go. Or buy yourself some clothes in the size you are aiming to become and promise yourself that you will be wearing them soon. Another idea is that if you are dying to eat fattening food – a cake, or thick bread and butter – allow yourself this treat. Serve yourself with the maximum of ceremony – you will probably discover that it isn't so marvellous after all. Anyhow it might prevent you from going on a binge.

5. COMPLACENCY

When you have lost a few pounds and are nearly at your target weight a feeling of complacency sometimes creeps in. Everyone is saying how well you look, that you really don't need to lose any more etc. Don't listen to them. Stick to your target. Go to a dancing class, go swimming – or have a massage.

6. BINGE EATING

'A hungry stomach has no ears.' French proverb

When dieting, most of us have an occasional overwhelming desire to stuff ourselves – to go on a binge. This is the time when you raid the kitchen and no food, however revolting, is safe from your searching mouth. When you feel this coming on, don't pretend you won't eat, and then pick the night away. Cook yourself a proper meal whatever the time of day or night, and eat it. Fill up on vegetables, carrots, celery, cabbage, cucumber, lettuce etc.

If you have a binge, don't despair and give up altogether by flinging yourself into an orgy of overeating. Don't punish yourself for being weak-willed – it happens to us all and really doesn't matter. Just go back to your diet with renewed vigour tomorrow.

7. COMPETITION AND ENCOURAGEMENT

If it is possible to diet with a friend, this will give you an added incentive. No one wants to lose face and give up, and we all want to lose as many pounds as, or more than, them if possible. By dieting with a friend it also means that you have someone to discuss things with – you can both moan and give each other encouragement. This is why the Weight-Watchers' clubs are so highly successful – they supply social pressure, competition and encouragement. For anyone with a tremendous amount of weight to lose, it is worth either joining a slimming group or making up your own small group with friends.

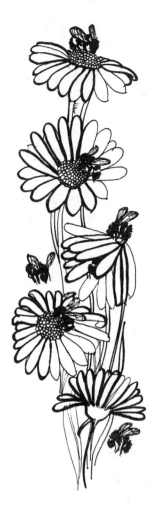

Helpful hints

I have been asking all my clients and in fact anyone whom I happen to speak to how they manage to lose weight. How do *they* stick to their diets, and what hints can they pass on? Here are the ones which emerged as the most useful:

1. HAVE A GOAL
Either work out a target weight, or buy a pair of skin-tight jeans that you want to be able to fit into – and sit down in!

2. DO YOU REALLY WANT IT?
Eat only when you are hungry, and *stop* the moment you are satisfied. This is incredibly obvious but to many of us it is more difficult than it sounds. Without thinking we shove food indiscriminately into our ever-eager mouths. Instead look at the food and ask yourself if you really want, or need it – no more gobbled handfuls or sneaked snacks.

3. PUT EVERYTHING YOU EAT ON A PLATE
This is particularly useful if you are a nibbler. You must put absolutely everything you want to eat on a plate before you eat it. So instead of simply breaking off a hunk of cheese and shoving it straight into your mouth, put it on a plate and then eat it. Similarly with those bread crusts, or that tablespoon of stew, those nuts or biscuits – before eating anything put it on a plate. You will get quite a shock. It is horrifying to see how much all this picking amounts to – just how much one actually eats without being aware of it.

4. RELAX BEFORE EATING
A client of mine who was very overweight went to a hypnotist. He taught her to relax and this helped her re-educate her eating. So often we eat, or smoke, because we are nervous. If you try and calm yourself down before you gobble up a plate of food you will find you can eat more slowly and enjoy it more. Simply sit down and calm yourself. If you are really het up and find it very difficult to relax, try some of the relaxation exercises on page 155.

5. EAT SLOWLY AND TALK A LOT
We all know that we should eat slowly but how many of us do? It's very difficult to break the lifelong habit of eating quickly, which often starts by mothers getting their children to 'hurry and eat up'. To break the habit of a lifetime's fast eating is extremely difficult, but if you want to be slim, indigestion-free and healthy, then you must try. Really taste all your food, ruminate over it. The slower you eat the less you will want.

As one was taught never to talk with one's mouth full – if you talk a lot, it is one way of making sure you eat less!

6. EAT ALL YOUR MEALS SITTING DOWN IN THE SAME ROOM
Be formal about your meals. Even if you are alone take your plate of food – even if it is only a lettuce leaf – sit down, preferably at a table and eat it in a civilized manner. If you are used to eating on the run, this is quite an education. I used to think it was a waste of time and would eat whilst doing something else. Don't – it's fatal. If you eat on

'*My beauty secret is to eat half of what is on my plate and not to drink at lunch.*'
Bette Davis

the run you just grab any food and swallow it down, whereas at a table you actually see what you are eating and in that way one eats infinitely less. When you've served yourself put all the extra food back in the kitchen – this will prevent you picking at it. If you then want a second helping you will have to get up to get it. In this way you will realize that you are having it!

7. THROW LEFTOVERS OUT

Some of us weak-willed, would-be dieters have a terrible habit – we eat sparingly and righteously at the table but once we get into the kitchen we turn into a monster waste-disposal unit. We 'tidy' everything up. We see that there aren't really enough leftover potatoes to keep and it seems 'such a pity to throw them out' that almost before we know what we've done, we've popped them into our mouth. *Don't*! Before you have time to think, throw all those odds and ends out, or, if you actually *will* use them up, put them away quickly in a covered dish. You must cover the dish to prevent your sneaky fingers from picking later.

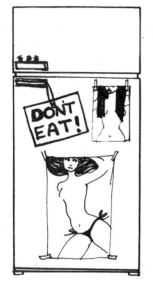

It's not terrible to throw food away – those starving millions really are not going to benefit from it anyhow – only your hips will!

8. NEVER EAT JUST BEFORE GOING TO BED

So often when tired we seem to get hungrier – with the tiredness, willpower goes and suddenly you feel like a late-night scavenger looking for tasty food. If this starts to happen to you, go to bed quickly – you're tired, not hungry.

It's bad for the digestion to eat heavily and then go straight to bed, as the metabolism does not work as efficiently, and it can make you fat. You should have 'the breakfast of a King, the lunch of a Prince and the supper of a Pauper'.

9. CON YOURSELF

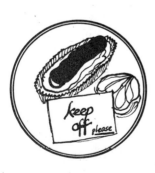

Convince yourself that you don't really like certain food. Instead of thinking of gorgeous gooey cakes as forbidden food (anything forbidden is instantly appealing) think of it as spot-making, starchy 'gluk' which is beneath your attention. You can put yourself off anything in this way.

10. SCATTER SLIMMING NOTES AND PICTURES EVERYWHERE

Put notes telling you to 'keep off', 'get thin', 'don't eat' etc. in all the key places. In the refrigerator, the biscuit tin, the drinks cabinet etc. Or if you don't like the school marmish notes, pin pictures of glamorous models in the appropriate places. My sister had a picture of an extremely glamorous model in the sweet tin. It was most off-putting. She just couldn't enjoy sweets having been reminded of how she hoped to look. Charts pinned on the wall in the kitchen are also useful reminders.

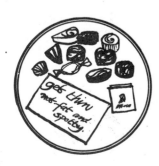

Sometimes it seems that the answer would be to put a lock on the kitchen door and keep out!

11. PRETEND THAT YOU ARE IN LOVE

One client has a novel way of losing weight. She realized that when she was in love she always got marvellously slim, and so now, whether

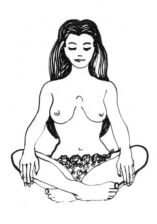

she is in love or not, she pretends that she is. She imagines that her heart throb is constantly with her, watching her every move. As she can't possibly let him see her gobbling down the children's left-overs, or gorging herself with rubbishy food, she says she automatically improves her behaviour; she cuts out all her secret eating and consequently she loses weight.

12. A WORD OF ENCOURAGEMENT

When starting on a diet, several clients have actually gained weight, and so I was delighted to discover the reason in Joseph Wederman's book, *Be Fit Not Fat.*

'*On a low calorie diet the loss of weight occurs in a staircase pattern. . . . First excess body fat is burned. About 4½ ounces of waters are formed and stored within the tissues for every ounce of this burned fat. Thus the dieter may not lose weight immediately, in fact he may gain several pounds for a brief period. But soon there is a change in the water tissue balance, the excess fluid eliminated and the scale shows a weight loss.*'

It is so discouraging to stick to a diet and not lose weight instantly. So if you ever find this, bear these facts in mind and keep persevering.

Calories

In any sort of diet, we come back ultimately to the basics of Calorie or carbohydrate counting – there really is no getting away from the fact if you consume fewer Calories than you use up, you will lose weight.

Calorie is the term used to indicate the amount of energy that may be released as heat when food is metabolized. As we all know some foods are very high in Calories and others are very low. As a general guideline fat yields more Calories – about nine Calories per gram – and proteins and carbohydrates about four per gram. In other words high energy food is high in Calories. The Calories of food equal Calories of energy, so if you are not energetic and eat more Calories than you expend, you store the excess as fat.

As a general rule a man needs about 3,000 Calories and woman approximately 2,000 Calories a day. If you cut down on your intake of Calories you *must* lose weight. A diet of 1,000 Calories a day sounds simple – so why isn't it? You have to re-educate yourself away from all your bad habits.

In order to use up 1 lb/450 g of fat you have to burn up 3,500 Calories. So, if you consume 1,000 Calories fewer than normal a day you will lose about 2 lbs/900 g a week. On the other hand, if you greatly increase your Calorie expenditure, you will also lose weight. But, unfortunately, you really do have to increase your output *greatly* to get any appreciable results. To use up 1,000 Calories you would have to play tennis or swim vigorously for at least four hours. To work off a large lunch you would have to play for at least seven hours, and even to get rid of one extra sandwich you would need to do vigorous exercise for about an hour! So it is rather impractical to think only of working off Calories – you have to decrease your intake as well.

That does not mean that exercise has no place in your diet – it has a *very important* place in our long-term plan for attaining positive health and slimness.

Too many people live sedentary lives. We ride in a bus or car instead of walking; we sit and watch television; we sit at desks in offices. If we increased our activity we would gradually lose weight – as long as we didn't eat any more! By doing only a little extra exercise we could easily lose about a pound a week. We could, and should, always do early morning warming-up exercises. We could also walk at least half the way to work and occasionally go swimming.

The more exercise we take the more Calories we will burn up and the *better* we will feel. As people get older they frequently become less active. The businessman will step straight into his car to get to work. The older woman tends to have a house filled with gadgets to make life easier – and less active! Inactivity definitely causes an increase in weight.

All this is written to try to make you aware of yourself and to try and goad you into activity (see the Exercise section on page 145).

Here is a rough guide to the number of Calories per hour we use up in the course of our daily lives.

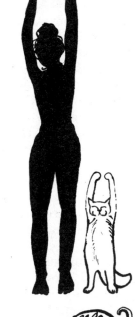

SEDENTARY ACTIVITIES   **60–100** Calories per hour
Sleeping
Thinking and day dreaming
Watching T.V.
Reading
Writing a letter

LIGHT ACTIVITY   **110–200** Calories per hour
Singing
Sewing or knitting
Ironing
Washing up
Typing

MODERATE ACTIVITY   **210–300** Calories per hour
House painting
Sweeping or scrubbing the floor
Walking slowly (2 m.p.h.)
Playing golf
Gardening
Making beds

STRENUOUS ACTIVITY   **310** +
Running
Walking fast
Gymnastic exercises
Swimming
Riding a bicycle
Skiing
Dancing
Walking up the stairs
Wrestling

One man's meat is another man's poison

More and more research is going into the interesting subject of food allergies. It has been found that the most varied of illnesses can sometimes be traced to food; from deep psychological disturbance and depression, to migraines, headaches, or just general aches and pains.

Under the supervision of a doctor, the patient is put on a monotonous diet of meat and either one fruit or one vegetable, for a week. Then other food is slowly added to the diet and the patient's pulse is taken before and after eating, to see if there is any adverse reaction. Gradually it is possible to establish which, if any, food someone is allergic to. The person can then either eliminate these completely from their diet or can sometimes be 'desensitized' to them by treatment.

According to the theory, it is quite common to be inordinately fond of, even addicted to, food to which one has an allergy. If you do not feel as well and fit as you would like, and do eat or drink a tremendous amount of one particular food, it might be interesting to go without it for a while and see if you feel any better.

For instance, caffeine is an addictive alkaloid, so if you drink a lot of coffee, you may be addicted to it. A research team in California tested 239 young housewives, and found that heavy coffee drinkers, given a drink with caffeine, felt better after it, while abstainers from coffee felt worse. In fact, heavy coffee drinkers (5–10 cups a day) found that they felt irritable and had withdrawal symptoms if deprived of the caffeine in their coffee. Dieters should take this into account, especially as in the diets I am asking you to cut out coffee altogether because I think that we all drink far too much. Replace it with a variety of herb teas.

We all have our own physical idiosyncracies – what is beneficial to some is harmful to others. Experiment with your peculiarities. Have you ever tried drinking lots and lots of water and seeing if you feel better? Unfortunately there is chemical pollution in water and some people are very sensitive to it. An alternative is to drink bottled water, although this can become very expensive. Why not buy a water purifier? I bought one recently and it has changed my life – my London water no longer has a vile taste and I now *enjoy* drinking water.

New things are constantly being discovered, so keep updating your information, and learn to experiment with your peculiarities. Try to work out your own personal balance.

Diet pills

Diet pills have been on the market for centuries. We all want the magic formula to whittle away our fat. If only these advertisements of the early twentieth century held any truth.

Here is an extract from an advertisement for Gordon Wallace's treatment headed 'Are you too stout?' (from *Secret Remedies*, 1912).

'If you are one of the thousands of much-enduring men and women who are unhealthily stout, or growing too stout . . . if your appearance is marred by a double chin or an ungainly bust, or a protruding abdomen, or any other disagreeable evidence of obesity here is an offer that will help you to remove the ugly defects in your physical appearance.

> *My method is unlike any other. I give my patients a true physiological treatment that restores lost Nerve Force and Nature does the rest.*
> *My treatment allows you to eat or drink whatever you like.'*

His packet of tablets, which were to be taken three times daily with food, when analysed, consisted of an extract and a vegetable powder. The extract was almost certainly bladderwrack, a common seaweed which contains a small quantity of iodine and was the basis of many of the nostrums for obesity. The vegetable powder was liquorice which has a slight laxative effect.

As for modern diet pills, I am against them – unless given under strict medical supervision.

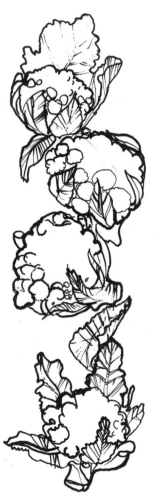

There are three types of diet pills. The ones you can buy over the counter are normally some form of laxative. They can give a very temporary weight loss but are not usually successful in long-term dieting. The second variety is prescribed by the doctor, and are usually amphetamine appetite suppressors. These pills stimulate your physical and mental activity and suppress your appetite. So you eat very little and yet feel very energetic (and frequently nervous). Although these pills do give an initial weight loss, this is usually regained very quickly once the pills are stopped. They can be addictive. As they do not *change* your eating habits, they are really only a short-term, rather risky and inefficient way of losing weight.

The third type of diet pills are diuretic pills, which are taken by people who think they are fat because they retain water. The diuretic pills increase their water loss. But these can be dangerous and again should only be taken under the strictest of medical supervision. Many women I know take them just before their period which is a time when more water is retained and which can cause tension. As a very short-term measure they can be of value but taken indiscriminately for weight loss they are both bad for you and ineffective. However, if you do take them you may need to take a supplement of phosphorus, as all the water loss can cause phosphorus deficiency. Eat lots of cauliflower if you do – it's very high in phosphorus.

Underweight

In this section on *Diet,* I have been writing principally about how to lose or maintain one's weight. But what about all those people who are underweight? To be too skinny can be as much of a problem as to be too fat.

First check with your doctor to be sure that there is nothing hormonally wrong with you, and then just eat as much nutritionally good food as possible.

The only positive advice I can give you is that you should learn to relax. Quite often underweight people tend to be very nervous and hyperactive. If you are able to relax and slow down, with any luck the pounds will slowly accumulate.

A preparation named *Sargol* was widely advertised at the turn of the century for the 'fattening' of persons who were too thin (*Secret Remedies,* 1912).

'This is an invitation that no thin man or woman can afford to ignore. We'll tell you why. We are going to give you a food that helps digest the other foods – a food that puts good solid flesh on people who are thin and underweight, no matter what the cause may be. A food that makes brain in five hours and blood in four – a food that puts the red corpuscles in the blood which every thin man or woman so sadly needs.

Chew one up with every meal, and in five minutes after you take the first concentrated tablet of this precious food it will commence to unfold its virtues, and it will by actual demonstration often increase the weight at the rate of a pound a day.'

These pills, when analyzed by the British Medical Association, were found to contain lecithin, hypophosphites of calcium, sodium, potassium, zinc phosphide, sugar, albumen, insoluble protein and talc and kaolin. None of which would be likely to produce the miraculous results claimed!

Crash dieting

'Trying to do something and failing is still better than trying to do nothing and succeeding.' Anon.

No one can form fat from anything but food and so if we wish to lose weight, *somehow* we have to take in less, and we must decide how to do this. Some lucky people only have to cut out the obvious starches and sugars and the pounds drop off, but for many of us it is not so easy. The fat simply will not budge and that is why faddy, crash diets are always so appealing. Between my clients and myself, I should think we must have tried every diet there is – living on nothing but bananas or grapefruit; on only liquids, or meat, or vegetables – you name it and one of us is bound to have tried it.

Although crash diets are very often scorned by doctors and nutritionalists, I believe that they can sometimes be useful. If by going on one of these diets someone who is very overweight loses a few pounds, this will encourage them to go on a long-term diet, and initial encouragement is very necessary for successful dieting. But all these quicky diets have the severe drawback of being only temporary measures. Their trouble is that they rarely give lasting results. You go on and off them, and the weight naturally 'see-saws' up and down. Not only does this fail to make you slim, but it can lead to food deficiencies. I even read that this constant 'on-off' dieting, with tremendous fluctuations in weight, could actually *increase* one's weight, and that it was one of the ways that farmers use to fatten up cattle!

So, crash diets are useful *only* if they do lead to a more soundly based, nutritionally sensible diet, which will re-educate you and your approach to food.

Each of us has an optimum weight when we feel just right – and it is this that we should strive to achieve – and maintain. The target is to find a diet that suits you and that you can stick to for life.

But before you embark on any sort of diet you must be in good health. If in doubt, don't hesitate to consult your doctor.

Fasting

This is the ultimate diet, when you take in absolutely no solid food and exist on water alone. If you are healthy, an occasional fast is thought to be highly beneficial as it revitalizes the digestive system by giving your body metabolism a rest. When fasting you have to drink as much water as you possibly can, at least four pints (2½ litres) daily, preferably mineral water. Surprisingly, after a day of fasting you don't feel hungry, but amazingly full of energy and well-being. It is quite safe to fast for two days but for any longer than that you should go to a doctor for medical supervision.

On a fast you can lose anything from two to four pounds (1–1½ k) a day depending on how overweight you are. When you return to normal eating you will find that you need less to fill you up.

Fruit juices only

This is not really fasting, but it has nearly the same effect on the body. You just lose weight a little slower – but it is infinitely easier to stick to. It is this that I have suggested we go on during the *Two-day blitz*. If you have never been on a liquids-only diet before, you honestly will find that it really is easy and that you will not feel hungry – whenever you feel the pangs of hunger just have a glass of mineral water. Some people are worried that they will feel tired but I have always found quite the contrary, and have been brimming over with health and energy. Try for yourself and see.

You can lose anything from 1–3 pounds a day and so on the *Two-day blitz* you should lose between 2–6 pounds.

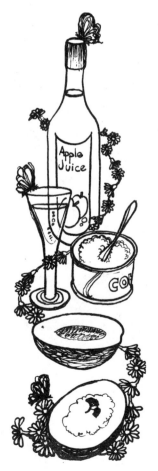

The high protein diet

Several of my clients swear by this diet, in which you eat nothing but lean meat, poultry, fish or eggs, for breakfast, lunch and supper. You may eat as much as you wish but absolutely nothing else. You must drink at least 8 glasses of water a day and as much black tea and coffee as you want. Never follow the diet for any longer than ten days.

Melon and cottage cheese diet

This is a lovely, easy diet to follow for a couple of days during a hot summer. At each meal you eat ½ a melon filled with 4 oz/100 g cottage cheese, and you drink a glass of pure apple juice. This combination is extremely filling and you can easily shed a few pounds. Only follow it for two days and again drink lots of water.

Eggnog diet

One friend swears by this diet, which again should only be followed for a couple of days. Mix together two eggs, two pints fresh milk, the juice of two oranges and one tablespoon olive oil. Mix all the ingredients together until they look frothy and light. This will provide you with about 5 glasses of 'Eggnog' which you drink to replace your meals. You may also drink as much herb tea (no sugar or milk), black coffee or water as you desire.

Food and drink

All this talk of abstinence, calorie counting, pills and crash dieting, can get a little upsetting. It will be quite refreshing to come across this section where I outline some food and some drinks which you can actually eat and drink without an acute dieter's conscience!

Yoghurt

Yoghurt enjoys the reputation of being a 'health food'. To an extent this is true, as yoghurt is rich in B vitamins and is a good source of protein (so too is milk from which it is made). The bacteria in yoghurt have a beneficial effect on the intestinal flora. If you have an upset, over-acid, stomach, yoghurt definitely helps to calm it down. However, many people buy fruit yoghurt which is loaded with sugar, in the belief that it is doing them good. This is very questionable as all that added sugar probably outweighs the good effects of the yoghurt bacteria.

Why not try making your own yoghurt – it is easy to make and tastes better than most commercial varieties. The secret of good yoghurt-making is to find a place where you can maintain a constant temperature of about 45°C (115°F). The ideal place is a warm airing cupboard, or on top of a storage heater, near the stove, or in a thermos flask. (Or you can use a commercial yoghurt-maker.)

Use any milk (skim if you are dieting and full fat if you are not). The milk must be sterilized and so you must boil it, unless it is Longlife or similar.

1. Bring 1 pint of milk to the boil.
2. Let it cool down to about 45°C. (I don't have a thermometer but if you can hold your finger in the milk comfortably for the count of 10 it is the right temperature.)
3. Put one tablespoon of plain commercial yoghurt into a wide-necked bowl (I use a glazed earthenware one) or a wide-necked thermos flask. Add the milk slowly and mix it evenly. Put the lid on the flask and leave it undisturbed or cover your bowl with cling film or a towel and place in your warm place of constant temperature.
4. After about 4–8 hours look at the yoghurt – if it has set it is ready. If not leave it for a little longer. When it is ready put it in the refrigerator so that it stops growing, otherwise it can become rather bitter. If you made it in the thermos flask pour it out into a bowl.

It really is incredibly easy. You have to experiment so that you get perfect results. If you like your yoghurt firm add a little powdered milk to it, or simmer the milk so that it contains less water. If you are not on a diet, and like it thick and creamy, try adding cream and my own favourite trick, half a jar of evaporated milk – that really makes it delicious, but very *fattening*!

Your home-made yoghurt has many uses. It can be eaten as it is, mixed with fruit, made up into salad dressing, or mixed with fruit juice to make delicious refreshing drinks.

Yoghurt drinks

Dilute your yoghurt with any fruit juice – yoghurt and apple or orange

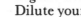

or tomato, or all three. Try mixing it with an egg and honey. In fact, mix it with anything that you can think of. It is fun experimenting and most combinations would be delicious.

Unfortunately yoghurt is quite high in calories (100 gm equals about 150 calories or 7 carbohydrates) and so these drinks should be taken as a snack or light meal rather than just a drink.

One way to cut the calorie count is by mixing with water, as in the following recipes:

LABAN

½ pt/300 ml yoghurt
½ pt/300 ml water
2 tablespoons finely
  chopped fresh or dried
  mint
salt

Everywhere in Turkey you see street vendors selling this deliciously refreshing drink. Beat the yoghurt and water together until they are thoroughly blended and then add in the salt and crushed mint. Serve chilled. It makes a lovely cooling summer drink to have with picnics.

You can also finely chop ¼ of a cucumber and add that to the *Laban*. This is also delightfully refreshing.

LLAHSI

Another yoghurt drink – this time thinned with rose water (the kind from the grocery shop, not the chemist) and mixed with honey. The honey, of course, means that the drink is slightly fattening but it has such an unusual, delicate flavour, I just had to include it.

Low calorie salad dressings

Whilst dieting you will be eating a lot of different salads and so here are some suggestions for salad dressings:

1. Wine vinegar or lemon juice, salt and pepper, garlic and a mixture of herbs.

2. ¾ cup of tomato juice, 1 tablespoon vinegar (cider), ½ teaspoon mustard, ½ teaspoon Worcestershire sauce, ½ teaspoon basil.

3. 2 tablespoons yoghurt, 1 tablespoon diet salad dressing, and ½ teaspoon lemon juice (optional).

4. 2 tablespoons yoghurt, Worcestershire sauce, garlic and herbs.

Drinks

If you drink a lot when dieting it curbs your appetite and makes you feel full. Water is obviously the ideal answer as it contains absolutely no calories. But even the purest, freshest water can become rather boring. So I have had great fun experimenting with drinks – working out recipes that are not only delicious but also very low in calories.

If you drink spirits the best piece of advice I can give you is to get a pub measurer – most of us over-estimate, and drinks become more and more generous, making the calorie intake leap up. So be sure to measure out your drinks – you will probably find that it also makes the bottle last infinitely longer!

When drinking spirits, the mixes add a large number of unnecessary calories – tonic water, ginger ale and coke are all horribly high in calories. Substitute low calorie mixes – and always read the labels to make sure that they *really* do contain no calories. Fruit squashes are also filled with sugar and terribly calorific, so buy low calorie squashes.

Make all your drinks look pretty, put them in your best glasses and garnish them with whatever seems appropriate – orange, lemon, cucumber or mint. Don't just gulp them down, sip and enjoy them.

DELICIOUS ELDERFLOWER DRINK

4 heads of elderflowers
(or 5 tablespoons dried
elderflowers)
4 pts/just over 2½ litres
water
Juice and rind of a lemon
1 tablespoon wine or cider
vinegar
6 sweetener pills (more or
less depending on the
sweetness of your tooth)

Mix all the ingredients together and let them infuse for 24 hours. Strain and then chill in the refrigerator before drinking. I think that this is one of the *most* delicious drinks, with a delicate fragrant taste, slightly reminiscent of lychees.

I was already singing the praises of this drink, when in an old herbal, I read that elderflowers were anti-spasmodic and diaphoretic (promotes sweating). They were also recommended for rheumatism, fevers and chills.

COLD GINGER TEA

Make a pint of strong lemon tea and to that add 1 teaspoon ground ginger, 10 cloves and sweetener to taste. Chill this in the refrigerator and either drink it by itself or better still, mix it with low calorie ginger ale. Garnish it with a slice of orange or lemon and sit back and enjoy it.

LEMON AND LIME COOLER

Mix lime juice (either fresh or low calorie lime juice) with the juice of half a lemon and dilute it with low calorie tonic water. This is incredibly refreshing. Garnish it with a slice of lemon.

JULAB

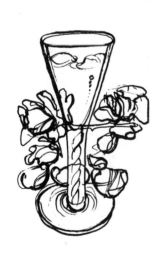

The word julep originally comes from this drink which is from the Persian *Gul* – rose and *ab* – water. It is made with rose water (the variety from an Indian delicatessen, not that from the chemist which tastes revolting). Mix the rose water with a teaspoon of honey (or a sweetening tablet) and a few raisins and pine nuts. Let it stand for about half an hour and then drink. To garnish float some rose petals in it to make it look really romantic.

CUCUMBER AND MINT

Liquidize half a cucumber and a sprig of mint. Add salt to taste. Strain it and dilute it with soda water. This is another delicious drink, as mouthwatering to look at as to taste.

SHARAAB HEALTH DRINK

Sharaab, the Arabic word which nowadays is usually used for an alcoholic drink, used to refer to this health drink which was drunk from Indonesia to Southern Spain. Mix 1 teaspoon of vinegar and a teaspoon of honey and dilute it with water. This gives you a tremendous lift and is, I find, especially good after fasting.

CHILLED FENNEL TEA

All the old herbals mention fennel for slimming. And so I make a large pot of this tea which tastes rather like anise, and drink some hot and then chill the rest. After it has been chilled it tastes rather like Pernod – absolutely lovely.

ORANGE SOUR

This is juice of an orange and a lemon mixed together and diluted with soda water. Sweeten to taste and garnish with a slice of orange and mint.

SPARKLING WINE CUP

Mix equal parts of wine and cold aromatic tea (Earl Grey or Jasmin). Into this put slices of orange, cucumber and mint (preferably lemon mint). Chill in the refrigerator. I further dilute it with soda water which makes it lovely and fizzy and rather like a poor man's champagne (about 20 calories a glass).

SLIMMING SANGRIA

1 bottle red wine
½ teaspoon cinnamon
Juice 2 squeezed oranges
3 oranges and 1 lemon, sliced
3 cloves
1 bottle soda water

Mix all the ingredients together, except the soda, which should be added after the other ingredients have been allowed to stand for a couple of hours. Served chilled, it is quite delicious.

The calorie and carbohydrate value of drinks

SOFT DRINKS

All measurements throughout are standard can or bottle sizes.

	Calories	Carbohydrates
11.5 fl oz can Coca Cola	140	33
11.5 fl oz can Dry Ginger	120	13
4 fl oz grapefruit juice	70	6
4 fl oz lemon juice	10	3
4 fl oz orange juice	70	15
4 fl oz tomato juice	25	5
11.5 fl oz tonic water	127	23

ALCOHOLIC DRINKS

All measurements are standard pub measurements.

	Calories	Carbohydrates
1 pt beer	170–414	40
⅙ gill brandy	75	20
⅙ gill Campari	115	30
4 fl oz champagne	90	20
1 pt cider, dry	208	53
1 pt cider, sweet	240	63
⅙ gill gin	55	13
⅓ gill port	190	20
⅓ gill sherry	70	15
⅓ gill vermouth, dry	110	15
⅓ gill vermouth, sweet	165	20
⅙ gill vodka	63	15
⅙ gill whisky	58	15
4 fl oz wine, dry	78	25
4 fl oz wine, sweet	89	28

The values on this chart are the average values. If you wish to be more precise use one of the pocket books with calorie or carbohydrate values.

Diet for the seven-day campaign

DAY ONE   Raw food day   (Total calories, 955)

	Calories
Breakfast	
The Health Cereal (see page 63) *or* 1 grapefruit and a slice of wholemeal bread	200

Lunch – main meal

LARGE RAW SALAD

For example: ¼ lettuce (10), ¼ cucumber (10), 1 medium carrot (10), sliced tomato (10), 2 tablespoons sliced cabbage (10), 4 radishes (5), watercress (5), 1 tablespoon chopped fennel (5)   65
+ 1 tablespoon sunflower seeds (and that's lots!)   170
1 piece fruit (apple, orange, pear, peach)   40
     275

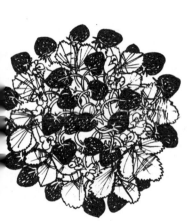

Supper – light meal

VEGETABLE AND SALAD MIXTURE

For example: 1 tablespoon chopped raw mushrooms (10), 1 chopped swede or a carrot (10), 1 chopped raw courgette (10), 1 tablespoon chopped onion (5), 1 tablespoon chopped sweet pepper (10), 2 or 3 florets raw cauliflower (10)   55
+ 2 tablespoons chopped almonds   60

FRUIT SALAD

For example: apple (40), orange (40), peach or strawberries (40) – anything but banana   120
1 small carton natural yoghurt   145
     380

Milk allowance (either ½ pt/300 ml skimmed or ¼ pt/150 ml whole)   100

DAY TWO   Raw food day   (Total calories, approximately 920)

	Calories
Breakfast	
The Health Cereal *or* 1 grapefruit and a slice of wholemeal bread	200

Lunch – main meal

4 oz/100 g smoked mackerel (an oily fish, rich in vitamins A and D)   240

or

3 oz/75 g steak tartare and 1 egg yolk (high protein and rich in vitamin B)   240

or

1 avocado pear | 240

+ salad of unlimited lettuce and watercress | 40

1 small carton low fat yoghurt, 1 tablespoon honey, with chopped fruit (e.g., 5 or 6 strawberries or 1 apple) | 200

480

Supper – light meal

1 enormous mixed chopped salad containing salad ingredients and vegetables and even fruit (extra 40), all mixed together | 100

Fruit, half melon or orange | 40

140

Milk allowance (either ½ pt/300 ml skimmed or ¼ pt/150 ml whole) | 100

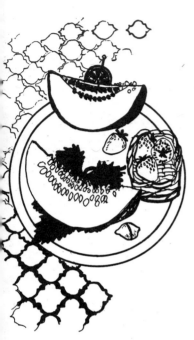

DAY THREE   Raw food day   (Total calories, 975)

Breakfast | *Calories*

The Health Cereal *or* 1 grapefruit and a slice of wholemeal bread | 200

Lunch – main meal

6 oz/150 g cottage or curd cheese (or 2 oz/50 g cheddar), mixed with fresh or dried herbs – chives, basil, pepper or garlic (filling and low in fat) | 240

+ ½ 8 oz/200 g tin pineapple rings preferably in natural juice (or pineapple pieces with syrup drained off, but add 20 calories more) | 70

+ watercress and lettuce salad | 10

Piece of fruit | 40

360

Supper – light meal

Salad of ½ cauliflower (50), 1 grated apple (40), and 1 table-spoon sultanas (25) | 115

Mix together with yoghurt and salad dressing and lots of freshly ground pepper and mixed herbs | 160

Piece of fruit | 40

315

Milk allowance (either ½ pt/300 ml skimmed or ¼ pt/150 ml whole) | 100

DAY FOUR   (Total calories, 935)
We are now going to include some cooked food but the calorie intake
is still very low.

Breakfast	*Calories*
The Health Cereal *or* ½ grapefruit, 1 egg (boiled or poached)	
+ 1 lightly buttered slice of wholemeal bread	200

Lunch – main meal

6 oz/150 g white fish – plaice or sole (light and easy to digest, and contains mineral elements). Bake in a medium oven wrapped in tin foil for 30 minutes	150
+ 4 oz/100 g green beans (no butter!)	20
+ 1 tomato and onion salad with basil	15
Fruit salad (see page 59)	140
	325

Supper – light meal

4 oz/100 g lean ham or tongue (protein)	240
+ 4 oz/100 g cooked leeks (or green salad of cucumber, green pepper and onion and lettuce)	30
Fruit	40
	310

Milk allowance (either ½ pt/300 ml skimmed or ¼ pt/150 ml whole)	100

DAY FIVE   (Total calories, 985)
Today is when you could invite a guest to lunch – they won't guess
that you are on a diet!

Breakfast	*Calories*
The Health Cereal *or* ½ grapefruit, 1 egg (boiled or poached)	
+ 1 lightly buttered slice of wholemeal bread	200

Lunch – main meal

Half a can chilled consommé and wedge of lemon	20
Baked joint of chicken (wrapped in foil with lots of lemon juice, salt and pepper: if you can find zeera – cumin seed – that's delicious added too). Bake in medium oven for about 45 minutes.	240
+ spinach and mushrooms (either cooked or raw as a salad)	50
+ tomato and onion salad with basil	20

BAKED APPLE

1 apple (approx. 6 oz/150 g) filled with 1 tablespoon sultanas and 1 teaspoon mixed spice (bake in medium oven for 40 minutes or until soft)	85

1 glass dry white wine	90
	505

Supper – light meal

Hard-boiled egg	85
+ large mixed vegetable salad	55
Fruit	40
	180

Milk allowance (either ½ pt/300 ml skimmed or ¼ pt/150 ml whole)	100

DAY SIX   (Total calories, 950)

Breakfast — Calories

The Health Cereal *or* ½ grapefruit, 1 egg (boiled or poached) + 1 slice lightly buttered wholemeal toast	200

Lunch – main meal

Grilled herring (approximately 4½ oz/110 g), containing essential fatty acids and vitamins. Grill for about 10–15 minutes per side	200

or

4 oz/100 g grilled steak	200
+ salad of lettuce, cucumber, chicory and watercress	65
+ 2 pieces celery or 2 tomatoes	20
2 pieces fruit	80
	365

Supper – light meal

2 oz/50 g Edam cheese or 4 oz/100 g cottage cheese	180
+ salad of watercress, bean sprouts and 1 green or red pepper	65
Piece of fruit	40
	285

Milk allowance (either ½ pt/300 ml skimmed or ¼ pt/150 ml whole)	100

DAY SEVEN   (Total calories, 975)

Breakfast — Calories

The Health Cereal *or* ½ grapefruit, 1 egg (boiled or poached) + 1 slice lightly buttered wholemeal toast	200

Lunch – main meal

4 oz/100 g grilled liver and kidney (vitamins A and D, and rich
    in *iron* – which if taken with orange is more easily assimilated
    by the body). Grill for about 10–15 minutes   195

or

1 lean lamp chop (grill for 5–10 minutes each side)   195

+ salad of 1 orange, 1 onion and bunch of watercress   70

Piece of fruit   <u>40</u>

    <u>305</u>

Supper – light meal

RATATOUILLE

1 small aubergine, green pepper, onion, tomato, courgette and
    garlic + 1 tablespoon oil. Slice and put in an ovenproof
    dish and bake in a medium oven for a good hour (or until
    the mixture is a soft, rich mass).   225

1 small carton natural yoghurt *or* 4 oz/100 g cottage cheese   <u>145</u>

    <u>370</u>

Milk allowance (either $\frac{1}{2}$ pt/300 ml skimmed or $\frac{1}{4}$ pt/150 ml
    whole)   <u>100</u>

MY HEALTH CEREAL

When you are on a diet it is extremely important to eat a good
nourishing breakfast, as this will prevent you 'picking' throughout
the morning. Ideally, you should have, 'The breakfast of a King,
the lunch of a Prince and the supper of a Pauper'.

    For breakfast each day you are allowed 200 calories. There is
a choice of either a cooked breakfast or my special breakfast cereal.

		calories	
3 tablespoons wheatgerm	100 ⎞		
1 tablespoon brewers' yeast	20 ⎟	150 ⎞	
1 teaspoon lecithin	25 ⎟		200
1 tablespoon bran	5 ⎠		
+ fruit juice, yoghurt or milk	50	50 ⎠	

Mix all the ingredients together and moisten them with yoghurt,
orange or lemon juice, or some of your milk ration. I have even
eaten it with water alone, and it still tastes delicious.

    I made up this cereal recipe when I was feeling particularly
tired. It was the middle of winter and I was reading all the books
on nutrition that I could lay my hands on and they all said how
important it was to have a nourishing breakfast. I decided to have
liver, eggs and toast each day, but somehow it was impossible: the

intention was there but I was always in too much of a hurry. And so I devised this cereal which is loaded with protein, minerals and vitamins, and takes only minutes to prepare.

Several of my clients also became converted to the 'Health Cereal' and we all swear that it makes us feel more energetic. It also tastes delicious, a lovely nutty flavour. The only ingredient that some people do not like is the brewers' yeast. I admit it is an acquired taste and if you *cannot* acquire it then take 6 brewers' yeast tablets daily instead. Swallow them down quickly and you won't taste them.

'Through the teeth
And past the gums,
Look out stomach,
Here it comes.'

Traditional American rhyme

'Imprisoned in every fat man is a thin one signalling wildly to get out.'

Cyril Connolly

'Sure check your lower limbs in pants
Yours are the limbs my sweeting,
You look divine as you advance –
Have you seen yourself retreating?'

Ogden Nash

'Praise is the best diet for us, after all.'

Lady Holland, *Memoir*, Rev. Sydney Smith

The Seven-Day Campaign

After the *Two-day blitz* you should be in just the right mood to continue on a diet and to take yourself really in hand.

I don't expect you to spend all your time beautifying yourself. That would not only be impracticable, but also terribly boring. I am assuming that, like most of us, you are busy and that you are going to squeeze this campaign into an already full life. If you have time on your hands, however, then you are lucky – you can spend even more time than I suggest and do everything at a more leisurely pace.

One of the benefits of a visit to a commercial health farm is that it changes your habits. Just as on holiday, you have a complete change of environment and routine. During this seven-day campaign try and do the same – change your habits and break out of the rut that we all so easily get into.

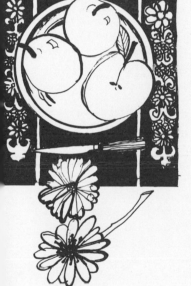

If you are usually inactive make sure that you do some form of activity – a swim or a walk – each day. If you are usually rushing from place to place, take it easier this week. Slow down and find time to read a book. If you usually go to the pub – go to the pictures. If you usually eat bacon and eggs – eat fruit. Try and change whatever habits you can – the stimulation will make you feel better and more alive. I am sure that the secret of a happy life is a balance of both routine and change.

Variety and stability are the key to happiness!

As with the *Two-day blitz* it will be more fun if you can persuade a friend to join you on the *Seven-day campaign*. You can then massage each other, help each other when experimenting with making cosmetics – and keep each other on the diet!

'What's the difference between an attractive woman and an unattractive one?' 'About an hour a day.'
Anon.

Each day of the *Seven-day campaign* is divided up into morning and afternoon (if you are at work, before and after work). I expect you to do about fifteen minutes each morning (longer if you can) and an hour each afternoon. I have only allocated this small amount of time because I thought that you actually might manage to do that, whereas if I expect you to do hours and hours, you might end up doing absolutely nothing.

So, let us start on our seven-day campaign.

Day one

Today you are on a Raw Food Diet (see page 59 for details). I chose this for several reasons: because it clears the system and skin; because you probably do not usually eat this type of food (the change element); and also so that you do not have to spend hours cooking, which could make you hungry.

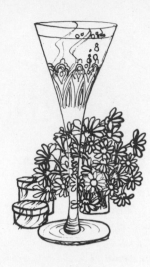

Morning

On waking have a large glass of cold mineral water. This is a marvellous way to start the day, making one feel more awake, and it tastes delicious.

Wash your face. This helps to wake you up. If you are one of those who never wash their face, then freshen it with skin tonic.

The mirror test

If you have just done the *Two-day blitz* then you obviously don't need to do this again. But if you skipped it before, please do the mirror test at the beginning of this campaign (see page 19).

Measure and weigh yourself.

Do your morning exercises. The standing ones (warmers) really do only take 5–10 minutes and so make sure that you do them today – and every day (page 147).

Cleanse, tone and cream your face. Make this into such a habit that you do it every morning (page 161).

Have breakfast (page 59).

Try and fit some form of exercise into your day. Either go for a long walk at lunchtime, play tennis, swim, go for a bicycle ride, or do an extra session of your exercises. Put on your favourite music and dance your way through the exercise section.

Afternoon/evening

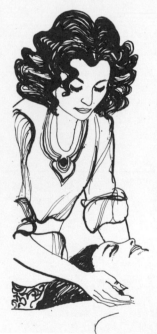

Body massage

Start the week by learning how to give a proper massage (page 81). You *can* massage yourself but it's infinitely easier if you are able to swop massages with a friend. Anyhow, one way or another, make sure that your body has a massage – to stimulate all those fatty areas, and pummel and knead them into an improved shape. Do not try and learn the whole body massage, just start on one area, learn the basic movements, and soon you will be able to do a whole massage.

After all that expended energy, you are probably in need of a lovely, long, relaxing bath. Herb baths fit beautifully into this category.

Baths

Herb baths have virtually died out, because everyone seems to find it easier to squeeze some bubble bath liquid (recipe, page 128) into the bath – but does it do as much good? Herbs have a tremendously beneficial effect on both the skin and one's mind – they are so aromatic. I have recently taken to having herb baths (I had to check all the recipes for this book!) and I find them marvellous. They have a delicate fragrance and leave the skin feeling really soft and smooth.

In a book written in 1665 with the lovely title of *Artificial Embellishments* there is this recipe: 'Take two handfuls of sage leaves, a little lavender leaves, roses and salt. Boil them and then bath in them. This is extremely softening to the skin.'

Practically any herbs or flowers can be used in your bath – just look around the garden and kitchen and take your pick. Amongst my favourites are lavender, rose petals and orange peel, for their soothing

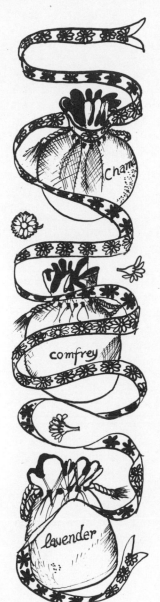

qualities and fragrance; chamomile and comfrey for their healing and emollient qualities; and rosemary and mint, because they are stimulating.

Mix a combination of these herbs together and store them in a large glass jar, where they are always ready to use. Put about 3–4 tablespoons into the bath. Don't just throw them in though: put them into a container of some sort otherwise you will have a lovely – but dirty – bath. In old recipes the herbs were always in little muslin bags. I use a metal container filled with holes which is really for cooking rice in. If you cannot find one of these (I found it in a Chinese shop) put the herbs into a little draw-string bag made from either muslin or any other loosely woven fabric. You can also use this to rub your skin with so that you get the full benefit of the herbs.

You could also try adding a couple of tablespoons of honey to your herb bath water. A spoonful of honey softens the skin, leaving it feeling like silk. It is also thought to relieve both tiredness and sleeplessness.

I always add a couple of spoons of honey to my herb bath – the more pampering the bath is, the better.

Day two
Another raw food day.

Morning

First have your glass of cold mineral water. Wash your face to wake yourself up. Do your exercises – by now you should be finding them easier – and enjoy all that stretching. It makes your body feel really alive.

Cleanse, tone and cream your face. And if you have any time left, practise the massage movements you learnt yesterday. Practise them on your thighs or hips, which can usually do with a little extra stimulation and attention.

Have breakfast (see page 59 for details of Day Two diet).

Afternoon/evening

Yesterday you concentrated on your body, so today I'd like you to study your face. Pull all your hair back and really study it in the mirror – an ordinary mirror, not a magnifying one. I hate magnifying mirrors because they're so depressing, showing up imperfections that, quite honestly, we don't need to see. No one but you is going to notice those tiny imperfections. It is the general impression that needs to be good: a clear skin that glows with health.

What is your skin type? (See page 161.)

Does your skin look as good as it should?

Do your eyebrows need trimming?

From today decide that you are going to begin giving your face the care it deserves. That means cleansing, toning and creaming at least once a day.

Having really studied your face, why not make some face cream with which to massage and pamper it?

Either choose a recipe from the *Skin* section starting on page 159, or make up this easy cream.

JASMIN ALL-PURPOSE CREAM

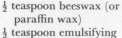

½ teaspoon beeswax (or paraffin wax)
½ teaspoon emulsifying wax
1 tablespoon almond oil
3 tablespoons rosewater
1 teaspoon glycerine
2 drops jasmin oil

Melt the waxes and oil together in a bowl in a water bath, and in a separate bowl heat the rose water and glycerine. Remove the bowls from the heat and slowly, stirring continuously, add the rosewater and glycerine to the oils. Continue stirring until it cools then add the jasmin oil. Do not stop stirring the cream until it thickens and sets. (I always use an electric beater on low speed to hasten the process.)

Glycerine, which is obtained from vegetable sources, is a humecant. This means that it retains moisture in the tissues and it also draws moisture up from the lower skin tissue to the surface. So a little is good, as in this cream, but if used too extensively, it can be drying.

These quantities give you about half a cup of lovely soft, fine cream which is quickly absorbed by the skin.

When I have been 'cream-making' I always give all the finished results to friends to test, and they voted this one of the very best. Use it under make-up, instead of make-up, as a hand cream, or a body cream – in fact use it anywhere and everywhere.

Isn't it fun! Now that you have made all that cream why not put it to use instantly and massage it into your face (see page 108 for the movements).

Day three

Today is the last day of the raw food diet. You should already be feeling thinner and more energetic.

Morning

Again the same routine, a glass of cold water, wash your face and then do your exercises.

Cleanse, tone and cream your face.

Have breakfast (see page 60).

Afternoon/evening

Do some extra exercises this evening, concentrating on your worst areas.

When you have completed your exercises and are feeling like a rest, lie down with your feet above your head. Better still, lie on a *slant board*, which is an instant reviver from mental fatigue. It is incredibly relaxing having all the blood rushing to the head: it nourishes the skin, and clears the brain. To make your own slant board, lean an ironing board against a low chair or bed, making sure that it is securely wedged, lie on it so that your feet are higher than your head and your body is at an angle. I lie on my slant board a lot, especially when I'm very tired or have a slightly aching back, and it instantly revives me. It is also the perfect place to relax when you've put on a face mask. Do try it.

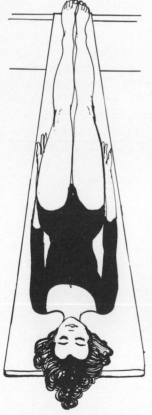

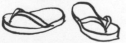

After relaxing on your slant board I thought you could tackle your body again.

Body scrubs

I am a great believer in scrubbing the body. If you want to have beautiful skin the best advice I can give you is to scrub your whole body each day with a string glove or loofah before having your bath. You only need to do it for a few minutes, but it improves the texture, removes dead skin and leaves the skin glowing with health.

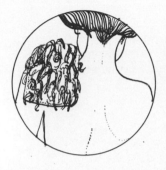

MAKE YOUR OWN STRING GLOVES

String gloves are sometimes quite difficult to find, and when I was in India I was taught an incredibly easy way of making them. Simply make up a square bag a little bigger than your hand, out of any tough material. Then sew bits of rough string all over it. Sew the string on anyhow and anywhere (an ideal job for a child just learning to sew!), so that you have a nice scratchy and rough surface.

SALT SCRUB

1 tablespoon sea salt
1 tablespoon kelp

Another way of giving your body a scrub is to massage it with kelp and salt. Mix these together, and rub your body all over with the mixture. This is a slightly messy procedure, so I'd recommend that you stand in the bath. Don't forget about those normally neglected areas – elbows, knees and feet. Massage them well with the mixture. (Incidentally, if you can't be bothered to scrub your body with the salt and kelp, put the mixture *into* the bath water instead – it makes for a very soothing and relaxing bath.)

When you have massaged your body thoroughly, and it is tingling with cleanliness, rinse all the salt off with warm water and apply a body lotion, concentrating again on your elbows, knees and feet. The following cream is ideal for use after the salt scrub – it is a rich body lotion, ideal for dry skin, for after too much sun, or for using when you practise your massage movements.

LAVENDER BODY LOTION

1 teaspoon beeswax
1 teaspoon lanolin
2 tablespoons petroleum jelly (vaseline)
5 teaspoons corn or peanut oil
4 teaspoons sunflower oil
2 tablespoons boiled water (or lavender water)
¼ teaspoon borax
¼ teaspoon lavender oil

Melt all the waxes and oils together in a bowl over a water bath. Dissolve the borax in the water in a separate bowl. Remove the oils from the heat and slowly, stirring continuously, add the water. Continue beating until it is cool and then add the lavender oil. This makes about 4 oz (100 g) of fine lotion which leaves the skin with a lovely sheen.

Culpeper said of lavender: 'Two spoonfuls of the distilled water of the flowers help them that have lost their voice, the tremblings and passions of the heart, and fainting and swoonings; applied to the temples and nostrils, to be smelt unto.' I also read that the Romans used to rub it on skin complaints, so if you suffer any of those afflictions,

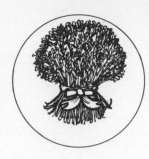

you had better rush to your lavender bushes.

(Lavender has yet another attraction – the dried flowers repel moths!)

Check your posture

Don't forget the 4 S's – string, shoulders, stomach and smile! (page 25).

As Chaucer said, 'Sweet as a flower and upright as a bolt.'

Day four

Morning

The usual early morning routine, of exercises and skin care.

One marvellous way to wake yourself up in the morning is to do some deep breathing. Stand in front of an open window and breathe in slowly and deeply.

> *'Deep breathing is an excellent exercise, and makes for the health which is the key to beauty. It should be practised slowly. The lungs should be extended as fully as possible, through the nostrils, not through the mouth, and the breath should be held until a slight feeling of discomfort is realized. The air should then be expelled through the mouth as slowly as it was inspired. Make the expulsion of air last as long as possible, then once again hold the lungs rigid, and do not inhale a fresh supply until discomfort again arises.'*
>
> *Invaluable Home References,* W. Foulsham

See page 61 for today's diet, your first on cooked food!

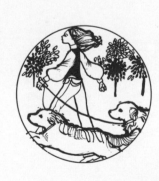

Afternoon/evening

Try and do some extra exercise today. Go for a long walk at lunchtime, jog around the block, do some of our exercises on page 151, or try skipping.

There is currently a craze for skipping in America and my jet-set clients will not go anywhere without their skipping ropes. They rightly say that it is one of the most perfect forms of exercise. It helps firm up flabby muscles, especially in the upper arms and thighs. It improves your posture and breathing and generally makes you feel marvellous. The lovely thing about skipping is that it is easy and terrific fun.

Depilatories

Tonight we'll look into depilatories and the question of hair on the legs. If you are a man, you are lucky as you don't have this problem, so just skip this section.

The question of hair on legs has always been a problem as we can see from this story about the Queen of Sheba.

> *'Jinns envious of Balkis (Queen of Sheba) so told Solomon that she had hairy legs so he had laid before his throne a pavement of crystal one hundred cubits square, then he had water poured on in so that when Balkis approached him she had to raise her petticoats as the water seemed to be of considerable*

depth. The only blemish were three goats' hairs which he removed with a compound of arsenic and lime, the first depilatory. (One of the five arts he introduced. The others were the act of taking warm baths, piercing pearls, diving and melting copper.)'

Legends of Old Testament Characters, Rev. Baring Gould, 1871

If your hair is fine and fair, I would recommend that you leave it alone. A little fine hair can look attractive but once you start 'de-fuzzing' it will be a continual problem. But for most of us de-fuzzing has to be a part of our regular beauty routine. We have to de-fuzz under our arms and on our legs.

The simplest method is shaving; the only criticism of this is that it has to be done extremely regularly, or you end up with prickly, stubbly hairs and legs like cactus plants. The alternative to shaving is waxing. In this method the hair is pulled out from the root and, depending on the speed of your growth, it only has to be done every 3–5 weeks. And when the hairs do grow again, they are not bristly.

For your initial waxing I would recommend that you go to a beauty salon, but once you see exactly how it is done, you can either do it yourself, or easier, get a friend in and wax each others' legs. Years ago an Indian friend gave me this recipe for wax – and it is still the best I have ever found.

1 lb 2 oz (500 g) sugar
juice of 2 lemons
1½ teaspoons glycerine
strips of cloth (e.g. from
    an old sheet)
or
strips of cellophane paper

Melt the sugar in the lemon juice and simmer very slowly until golden brown, cook it for 10 minutes and then remove from the heat. Add the glycerine and mix well.

Allow the wax to cool before using it – apply a little on the inside of your wrist to test it. You need to use the wax while it is as warm as possible but obviously you don't want to burn your legs.

Using a wooden spoon, apply the waxing in thin strips, going down from the knee towards the foot. Press the wax down and then put a piece of cloth or cellophane paper on top. Again press down and then taking the end of the strip, rip it towards you. Rip it off as fast as possible and all the hairs will come out with the wax.

At first it is slightly messy and difficult but, as with everything else, practise makes perfect.

A friend in California always uses this recipe and swears by it. With practise it is a relatively quick, extremely effective, easy method of hair removal.

You can also use this wax under your arms but for that it really is much, much easier if you can swop waxings with a friend.

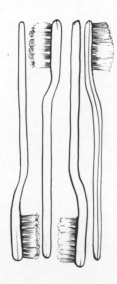

Teeth

Pearly white teeth are a tremendous asset to anyone in the search for health and beauty. Make sure that you go to the dentist at least every six months for a check-up. It is horrifying to learn that a vast number of people never go to the dentist, because they are afraid. This fear is totally unfounded. With all the modern equipment, a visit to the dentist need not be painful – especially if you go frequently. Prevention is better, and less painful, than cure.

2 tablespoons salt
3 tablespoons bicarbonate
  of soda

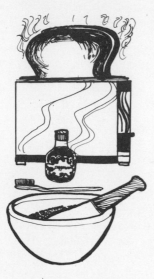

¼ cup boiled (or purified)
  water
1 teaspoon boric acid
1 teaspoon glycerine
¼ teaspoon tincture of
  myrrh

TOOTH POWDERS

One of the best tooth cleansers, a powder, is simple to make. If you brush your teeth with this simple mixture it will make your teeth beautifully white – it even removes nicotine stains! This basic mixture can be improved by the addition of 1 tablespoon of ground orange peel. This makes all the difference, as it tastes good and makes the breath smell sweet.

Another very good tooth powder can be made by burning a couple of slices of bread and pounding them into a fine powder. Add a couple of drops of peppermint to this and you have a marvellous toothpaste.

MOUTH WASHES

One of the problems about being on a diet is that your breath can begin to smell. So during your diet do take particular care with cleaning your teeth and try using these mouth washes – they are delicious. A very simple mouth wash can be made by diluting witch hazel with water, 1 part witch hazel to 10 parts water.

If you feel more adventurous, then here is another slightly more complicated mouth wash to try.

Dissolve the boric acid in the water and then add the other ingredients. Put the mixture into a bottle, shake them together and it's ready for use.

This recipe is adapted from one I was given in hospital, it has a disinfectant action, and tastes slightly bitter – if you find it too strong, dilute it further with water.

Anise seeds

In Afghanistan, when we had finished our meals, little bowls of anise seeds were brought around with the green tea. Chewing these seeds aids the digestion, relieves flatulence and sweetens the breath. Turner in his *Herbal* of 1551, says that 'Anyse maketh the breath smell sweeter and swageth payne'. It was also thought to avert the evil eye.

Cardomum

Chewing cardomum seeds is another way of sweetening the breath. They have a very refreshing taste.

Day five

Morning

Begin the day in the same way with your exercises and skin care. By now you should really be quite fit and so you could attempt to do what I consider the best beauty treatment in the world, the headstand. Try and spend about two minutes upside down, your head resting on a folded mat and your legs up against the wall. If you can manage to do a headstand you should do one every single day of your life. It is an instant beauty treatment – the blood rushes to your head, feeding the skin and keeping the facial muscles firm and young. But it is not only a beauty treatment, it is also the most marvellous reviver if you are feeling tired. It also helps clear the sinus and improve the circulation generally.

I cannot stress enough the virtues of the headstand – I could go on for hours why you should do one every day. If I had to choose only one way to help in the fight against age, I would choose the headstand. It is the cheapest, most priceless beauty treatment there is.

See page 61 for today's dietary advice.

Afternoon/evening

Today I thought we could pamper ourselves – and give ourselves a facial.

Having a facial is a wonderful experience, a real luxury treatment. It will ease out strain and any other tension lines from the face, leaving it looking, and you feeling, relaxed and refreshed.

Allow yourself about an hour. (It can be done in half an hour, but if you can relax and take an hour so much the better.) Make sure you will have absolute peace for the whole hour (try and organize the children etc. beforehand).

Ideally you will be swopping your facial with a friend, but if that is impossible the benefit your skin gets from the facial you give yourself is exactly the same – it just will not be quite as relaxing. Incidentally men too can enjoy having facials: there is nothing effeminate about men having facials as they suffer from headaches and blemished skin, and look much better with a good clear skin and a face devoid of tension.

Follow the same procedure if you are giving the facial to yourself or to someone else. First collect together everything you need: herbs, a bowl and towel for face steaming, cleansing cream, skin tonic, massage cream, cotton wool, face mask, eye pads.

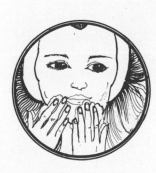

1. Tie your hair back and put on a scarf to protect it from the oils.

2. *Cleanse the face.* Apply cleansing cream. Really massage the cream in and remove all traces of dirt.

3. *Remove the cleansing cream.* Wipe off the cleansing cream with dampened cotton wool.

4. *Tone the skin.* Stimulate the skin by patting it with skin tonic. To do this really professionally use a 'patter'. You can easily make a 'patter' out of a 4-inch square of damp cotton wool. Fold the left corner over and then, starting with the right corner wrap it up – and there you are, you've made a 'patter'. Moisten the heavy tip with skin tonic, hold the other end and with a brisk slapping movement pat all over the face. The neck and chin greatly benefit from this, but avoid any area where there are broken veins.

5. *Massage the face.* Apply the cream or oil, and massage the face – stroke, pinch, stimulate and soothe. Follow the movements on page 108. Some people like to massage with cream and others with oil – try both and see which you prefer (recipes on next page).

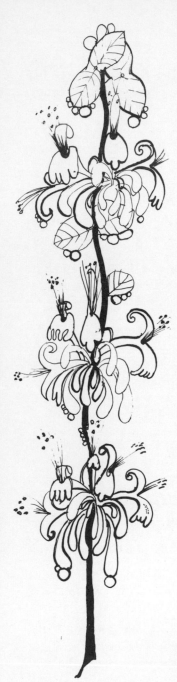

6. *Steaming the face*. The most thorough way of cleansing the skin is to steam it. It unclogs blocked pores and stimulates the circulation.

Add two tablespoons of herbs and flowers to a bowl of boiling water. Choose your herbs from the list on page 30 or use a mixture as suggested here.

(a) lavender, lemon peel, rosemary and thyme for their stimulating and antiseptic qualities.
(b) chamomile, comfrey, elderflowers and rose petals for their soothing and healing qualities.

Lean over the bowl with a large towel over your head so that you make a tent over the bowl. Keep your head about a foot away from the water. Steam the face for about 10 minutes and then wipe it with dampened cotton wool.

7. *Tidying up the face*. In other words, trim your eyebrows and if you have any blackheads that you cannot resist, now is the time to extract them – when the skin is softened so that they come out easily. Always use a fresh piece of cotton wool to do the extraction and then dab it with some skin tonic. Do not force blackheads out, undue pressure will mark the skin.

8. *Apply a face mask*. Again wipe the skin with skin tonic and then apply a mask (see page 170 for some mask recipes).

9. *Put on eye pads*. Soak two tea bags, put them on your closed eyelids and *relax*.

10. *Remove the mask*. After about fifteen minutes remove the mask with warm water.

11. *Apply light cream*. Massage some more cream into the now beautifully clear skin. Use a light cream and leave the skin without any make-up (it won't need it). Your face will be glowing with health and looking beautiful.

You will need to use either some massage cream or oil for your face massage and so here are some recipes.

ALMOND MASSAGE CREAM

Melt all the waxes and oils together over a water bath. When they are melted, remove from the heat and slowly, stirring all the time, add the water into which you've dissolved the borax in a separate bowl. Beat until the cream cools and thickens, using either a clean wooden spoon or lowest speed on a kitchen mixer.

This cream has a low melting point which means that it becomes lovely and soft with the heat of the skin – and that makes it ideal to use for massaging.

I have added a drop of almond oil to make it smell of almonds, which is always popular, but obviously you can add whatever perfume you happen to prefer at the moment. Honeysuckle oil is always a great favourite with my clients.

½ tablespoon beeswax
3 tablespoons coconut oil
2 tablespoons almond oil
1 tablespoon sunflower or wheatgerm oil

4 tablespoons boiled water
½ teaspoon borax

1 drop almond essence

You may prefer to massage with oil and so here are two lovely recipes.

SANDALWOOD FACE OIL

2 tablespoons almond oil
1 teaspoon wheatgerm oil
2 drops sandalwood oil
1 drop jasmin oil

Simply mix the oils together in a bottle, shake and use. This is a lovely, superfine face oil which is ideal for use when massaging.

It is highly aromatic due to a combination of sandalwood and jasmin – an exotic oriental and sophisticated smell. Unfortunately all vegetable oils eventually go rancid, but wheatgerm oil being an anti-oxidant does help prevent that. It is also vitamin E which has a tremendously beneficial effect on the skin.

FRAGRANT FACIAL OIL

2 tablespoons almond oil
1 teaspoon wheatgerm oil
3 drops rose geranium oil
2 drops orange blossom oil
1 drop honeysuckle oil

Again mix all the oils in a bottle and shake them together. This oil has a lighter flowery fragrance.

Day six

Morning

Again start the day with the same routine; a glass of cold water, your daily exercises and cleansing, toning and creaming your skin.

Scrub your body with a loofah and then massage it when you apply your body lotion.

Today is 'hair-washing' day, which makes it the perfect day to go swimming first. Really swim energetically. Try and do at least ten lengths, going as fast as you can.

See page 62 for what you can eat today.

Afternoon/evening

Conditioning the hair

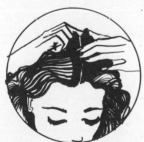

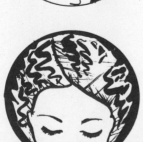

Most hair can do with conditioning. The easiest conditioner is oil – olive or coconut – which you simply massage into the scalp and hair.

First heat the oil, then make partings all over your head, apply it to the roots, and massage it into the scalp. Move your scalp about and try to loosen it, work with firm rotary movements all over the head. Then, with the tips of your finger-nails, make a fast scratching movement to stimulate the blood and bring it to the surface. A Pakistani friend taught me this way of massaging the head and her head massage is far better than any I have ever had at a hairdressing salon. She told me that when she was a child she used to massage her father's scalp and that he would say that he wanted to feel the oil coming out through his eyes!

When you have thoroughly massaged the oil into the scalp and your head is tingling, wrap your head up to keep in the heat and help the absorption of the oil. The traditional way of doing this is to wrap it in warm towels but I find it much easier to use silver kitchen foil (the silver turban also looks rather attractive!).

The oil should be left on the hair for about half an hour and so during this time do some *exercises*.

Put on your leotard and your favourite music and dance your way through the exercise section.

All that exercise should have made you hot and some of the oil should have been absorbed into your hair, so now wash it out.

Shampooing the hair

It is possible to make one's own shampoo with green soap but my attempts have never been very successful. Instead I use any commercial shampoo and enrich it by adding an egg.

PROTEIN RICH SHAMPOO

1–2 tablespoons shampoo
1 tablespoon water
1 egg

Beat the egg, water and shampoo together which makes it frothy and very easy to use. Wash your hair and rinse it thoroughly. As with washing your face, it is extremely important to get rid of all the soap. Carry on rinsing until your hair squeaks when you squeeze out the water.

Give it a final rinse with either diluted vinegar if you are a brunette, or diluted lemon juice if you are a blonde. This final rinse helps to remove the last traces of soap and to restore the acid mantle to the hair.

The important thing to remember when washing your hair is to treat it with care. When it is wet the hair is very vulnerable, becoming very stretchy, and is easily broken. A friend who has been trying to grow her hair down to her waist tells me that it has improved considerably since she followed the advice given her by a model who never brushes her hair after washing it, until it is completely dry. Apparently it's not the expected mess of tangles, so is definitely worth a try.

HOW TO TIE A TURBAN

This is not essentially anything to do with beauty, but turbans are such incredibly useful things that I feel they should be mentioned. Although turbans have been fashionable (on and off) for years, very few people know how to tie them.

The marvellous thing about turbans is that they cover up a multitude of sins. They are a 'life saver' in emergencies; if you are going out and your hair needs washing, they not only disguise the fact but they also make it look as though you've made an extra effort. If you oil your hair and want to leave it on all day, with a turban on, no one will know.

A turban adds the finishing touch to any outfit.

There are obviously hundreds of ways of tying them. I will show you one and then it is up to you to experiment.

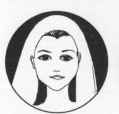 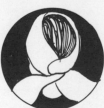 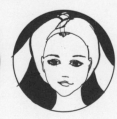 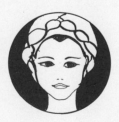

Day seven

Morning

Begin the day in the usual way – a glass of delicious, cold fresh water. Then do your exercises which you must be finding very easy by now, so don't forget to do either a head- or shoulder-stand, or, if you can't manage them, lie on your slant-board with your feet higher than your head.

Having finished your exercises, wash, clean, tone and cream your face and apply your body lotion (see Day Three, page 69).

See page 62 for your last day's food.

Afternoon/evening

Fit some form of exercise or sport into the day – go for a long country walk, play tennis or do a really long exercise workout. Put on your leotard and your favourite music, and enjoy yourself by exercising to the music.

Today I thought you should check your hands and feet, and give yourself a manicure and pedicure.

Hands

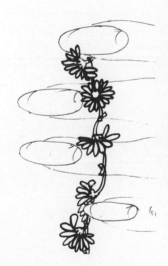

Your hands are a tremendous give-away – they can almost instantly tell someone your age and occupation, and through the nails – your state of health. There is usually very little fat on the upper hand and the palms have no sebaceous glands which makes them one of the driest parts of the body. And so your hands can, all too easily, become lined and wrinkled. To prevent this you really should wear rubber gloves to protect them from water and detergents, and protective hand creams to protect them against the sun and wind. In fact, use hand cream lavishly, and apply it each time you wash your hands. Keep jars of it everywhere – near the telephone, next to the wash-basin, in your handbag, next to the bed – and apply it whenever you remember. Your hands need *constant* pampering.

Massage is terrific for the hands, as it exercises them, and all the oil and cream you use lubricates them – yet another reason to learn to massage!

Here is a recipe for a very simple, yet very effective hand cream.

NON-GREASY PROTECTIVE HAND CREAM

1 tablespoon emulsifying wax (or lanette wax SX)
2 teaspoons cod liver oil
¾ cup boiled water
essential oil (lemon or orange)

Simply melt the wax and heat the oil over a water bath. Remove from the heat and slowly, stirring all the time, add in the warm water. Continue stirring until it starts to set (that will be fairly quickly) and then add a few drops of essential oil.

Although we have gone through the procedure for a manicure (see page 28), not everyone has nails that they consider are really worthy of being manicured. Their nails always seem to break and split.

Here are some hints on how to improve them. If you take 1 table-

spoon of gelatine daily for three months you should notice an improvement. In hospital tests they discovered that this restored normal
appearance and prevented nail brittleness. One researcher found that
ridged, furrowed nails were cleared up when vitamins A, B and D
were taken, and so why not check the nutrition section for food rich in
these vitamins and try to add them to your diet.

Buffing and massaging cream into the nails also helps growth, and
strengthens the nails. The following nail cream contains all the
ingredients I could think of that are good for strengthening the nails.

NAIL AND CUTICLE CREAM

1 tablespoon lanolin
2 teaspoons beeswax
1 tablespoon petroleum
  jelly
½ teaspoon almond oil
½ teaspoon castor oil
½ teaspoon cod liver oil

1 tablespoon boiled water
¼ teaspoon gelatine
¼ teaspoon glycerine
¼ teaspoon borax

Melt the oils and waxes together over a water bath. In a separate bowl
dissolve the borax and gelatine in the water and glycerine. Remove the
oils from the heat and slowly, stirring all the time, add in the warm
water. Continue stirring until it sets.

This cream is a very rich nourishing cream which you should use as
frequently as possible. These quantities make about half a cup. Use
it really lavishly, and it will do wonders for your nails.

EASY CUTICLE CREAM

2 tablespoons petroleum
  jelly
½ teaspoon glycerine
drop of red food colouring

Beat all the ingredients together and you will have an instant cuticle
cream which is almost identical to many that are on the market.
Really nothing could be easier than this, so do make – and use – either
this or the previous cuticle cream, *frequently*.

Although I am encouraging you to grow your nails, beware of
extremes. Nails should not be too long as is demonstrated by this
anecdote: 'An English lady, writing to a relative about meeting the
Dowager Empress of China said: "One by one we were presented to
the Dowager Empress, and when I took her extended royal hand her
fingernails were so long that it was like shaking hands with a bundle
of pencils."' (From *The Dragon Empress* by Marina Warner.)

Just before you do your pedicure, pamper your face by putting on a
face mask. Choose one from the mask section (page 170), and leave it
on while you do your pedicure.

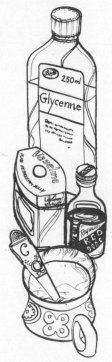

Pedicure
As you have learnt how to give yourself a professional manicure, a
pedicure presents no new problems. You follow exactly the same routine.
To recap:

1. Remove old varnish.

2. File or cut toe nails.

3. Apply cuticle cream and gently push the cuticles back.

4. Massage the feet with oil or cream.

5. Soak your feet in a bowl of warm, soapy water and scrub the oil
off your toe nails.

6. Dry your toe nails and buff them.

7. Before applying the varnish put little wads of cotton wool between each toe. This prevents you getting nail varnish on the next toe, avoids smudging, and altogether makes the job much easier.

8. Apply base coat, a couple of coats of nail varnish and top coat.

And there you are – your feet should look as beautiful as your hands.

Look back at your progress during the last week.
   Weigh and measure yourself. You should have lost either (or both) weight and inches and be looking and feeling slimmer and healthier.
   Are you remembering to drink plenty of water?
   Have you done your exercises every day?
   Is your hair beautifully shiny?
   Are you altogether well groomed?
In other words, have you kept (more or less) to the *Seven-day campaign*?
   Hopefully the answer is yes, and by now you are filled with energy and enthusiasm which will take you on to do the *Three-week health kick*.

> *'See! How she leans her cheek upon her hand:*
> *O! that I were a glove upon that hand.*
> *That I might touch that cheek.'*
>
> *Romeo and Juliet*

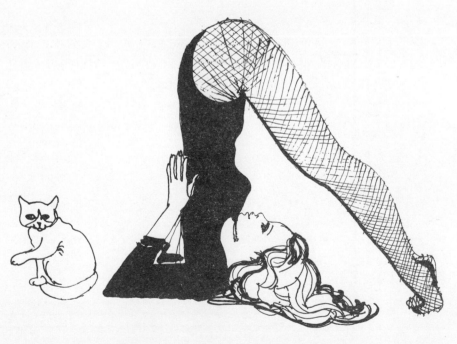

7-day campaign – quick check list

	Morning	**Afternoon/evening**
DAY 1	*Raw food day*	
	Mirror test	Body massage
	Exercises	Herb + honey baths
	Cleanse, tone and cream face	
DAY 2	*Raw food day*	
	Exercises	Study your face
	Cleanse, tone and cream face	Massage your face
	Practise massage movements	Make all-purpose cream
DAY 3	*Raw food day*	
	Exercises	Exercises
	Cleanse, tone and cream face	Slant board
		Body scrubs
		Make lavender body lotion
		Check your posture
DAY 4	*1,000 calories*	
	Exercises	Exercise (skipping?)
	Cleanse, tone and cream face	Depilatories – make wax
	Deep breathing	Teeth – make tooth powders and mouth washes
DAY 5	*1,000 calories*	
	Exercises	Give yourself a facial
	Cleanse, tone and cream face	Make massage cream and face oils
	Headstand	
DAY 6	*1,000 calories*	
	Exercises	Hair day. Conditioning massage
	Cleanse, tone and cream face	
	Scrub body	Exercises
	Swimming at lunch	Shampooing
DAY 7	*1,000 calories*	
	Exercises	Exercise
	Head stand	Weigh and measure yourself
	Cleanse, tone and cream face	Give yourself a manicure and a pedicure
	Body lotion	Look back at your progress

Massage

Massage is very easy. It is simply an extension of something that we do already: when we hurt ourselves we rub the sore area; we stroke our foreheads when we have a headache; we pat a child on the back or the head to reassure it; and we stroke our pets.

In many parts of the East everyone from the youngest child to the oldest grandparent knows how to massage, and I think that is something we ought to emulate. We don't all want to be experts and give full body massages, but just to know how to soothe an aching leg or rub someone's shoulders is valuable. Even a little massage can make the recipient feel so much better. Massage is one of the most useful of accomplishments; it can give so much pleasure for so little effort. I asked some students from my massage courses to tell me how they had found it. They all practised massage away from the classes – and in many different ways. Several used it at work, rubbing their colleagues' shoulders after a busy day over a desk; others after any form of sport. One woman massaged her son to sleep; another relaxed her tense husband. One found it the perfect way to repay hospitality when travelling and staying with people. Another refreshed his child and housework-weary wife with it, and yet another found it helpful when rubbing down his horse!

Massage has been practised throughout history – there are records of it being used by the Egyptians, the Greeks, the Romans, the Chinese and the Japanese. Although the terminology is sometimes different, their methods seem very similar and have remained so to this day.

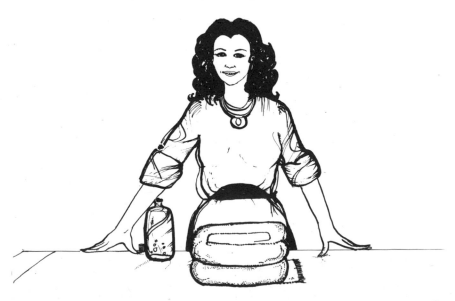

What is massage?

The word massage, which means to knead, describes the manipulation of the soft body tissue with the hands. The movements can be either soothing or stimulating.

It affects the local and general lymphatic and circulatory systems, increasing the superficial blood circulations and bringing blood to the skin and muscles. This alone makes you feel more awake and alive.

It affects the muscular and nervous system; releasing tension and hindering fibrositis. It relaxes the voluntary muscles and helps them to maintain their best possible state of nutrition and flexibility, so that they can function at their maximum. It is for this reason that footballers, boxers and other sportsmen have massage.

And most important: it makes you feel cared for, and gives a tremendous feeling of well-being.

What do you need?

Really only your hands. Your hands need to be firm but relaxed. This may sound like a contradiction of terms, but although slightly difficult at first, it will soon become easy. Let your hands mould around the contours of the body. Use the whole of your body to give you rhythm and strength. This stops you from straining and tensing your arms and hands, and prevents you from getting exhausted.

Relax your hands by shaking them vigorously before you begin and warm them up by rubbing them together. People do not like massage with cold hands, except perhaps in very hot countries!

Before you start a massage, release the tension from your arms and hands by doing this easy exercise.

Stretch your arms out to the side, with your palms turned down. Bend your hands back from the wrist, hold them there for a second and then bend them right down. Flap them up and down in this way several times. This sounds too simple, but you'll be surprised at how much it relaxes your hands.

Oil

Although it is possible to do a massage without using any form of lubrication, I find that oil makes it much easier and more enjoyable.

You can use either vegetable, mineral or baby oils. I like to use vegetable oils as these go into the skin, whereas mineral and baby oils don't, and tend to block the pores. The most commonly-used vegetable oils are sunflower, corn, olive, almond, safflower and avocado oil. My favourite is almond oil which is very fine, but also rather expensive, and so I sometimes mix several oils together. Most oils tend to have a rather heavy, even rank smell, and so they can be greatly improved with the addition of some essential oils.

No. 1
$\frac{2}{3}$ cup almond oil
$\frac{1}{3}$ cup sunflower oil
4 drops jasmine oil
8 drops rose oil

In both recipes, just mix all the ingredients together. In the second recipe, honeysuckle or orange-flower oil could be used instead of lavender.

No. 2
¾ cup safflower oil
⅓ cup corn oil
10 drops lavender oil
2 drops camphor

These recipes are just suggestions; experiment with all sorts of essential oils; mix your favourites together to get your own individual scent – and mix them beforehand, to give the scents time to blend. Like good wine they improve with time! Some people like to massage with powder, but I find this more difficult, and it dries the skin. Also, you don't have the advantage of all those lovely scents we have with oils.

Keep your oil in a plastic bottle which has a narrow opening – an old hand-lotion or shampoo bottle is likely to be ideal. These narrow-topped bottles make life easier, for two very practical reasons. The first is that, at some time, you're bound to knock over the bottle, and oil is difficult to get out of carpets and blankets; but with a narrow opening, hopefully you will only spill a drop.

The other reason is that to give a really good, flowing massage, you need to keep your hands in constant contact with the body, but every now and then you may need to apply more oil. The way to do this is to keep one hand on the body, and with the other pour some oil onto the back of that hand. This sounds unnecessarily complicated but is actually easy to do and in this way you can maintain the flow of the massage. This also ensures that when the oil touches your friend's body it will already be slightly warm. It is horrible to have oil poured straight onto the body; it feels cold and slithery. So always apply the oil to your hands first. Rub them together and stroke on the then slightly warmed oil.

Where to massage

A table

It is of course ideal to have a massage table but if, like most people, you have not got one, the next best thing is a large, steady table.

The table needs to be high enough to come to the top of your thighs, so that when standing up straight, the palms of your hands just touch the top. It must be long enough for your friend to lie on without hanging over the edges! With luck your kitchen or dining-room table will be suitable. Pad the table with a couple of blankets so that it doesn't feel too hard and uncomfortable.

The floor

Although I have a massage table, I rarely use it, as I find it easier to massage on the floor. Some people think this awkward and tiring but I like the firmness and all the space around me. By kneeling or sitting you can move around the body easily and put the weight of your body into the massage which makes it less tiring. Again you will need to pad the area to make it comfortable for your friend.

One word of warning; if you do massage on the floor, remember to kneel on something soft. I never bothered to do this, until one day as I walked downstairs wearing a beautiful, long silk dress, I heard a loud scratching sound. It was my calloused knees catching on the fine silk!

Your bed

Most beds are too soft for giving a good massage. All your strength will disappear into the mattress. So, unless the bed is very hard, or you are extremely strong, I do not advise it; however, if you are giving a very soft, gentle massage, it is possible, if the bed is very low, to kneel at the side, so that you do not strain your back.

Their comfort

To sum up, the most important thing when giving a massage is to make sure that both you and your friend are comfortable. Try massaging on different surfaces and see which you find the most convenient. Once you have chosen the place, pad the area with a doubled blanket covered by a sheet. Also, make sure that you have two or three large towels to keep your friend covered up and warm. It is surprising just how cold it can be when you're being massaged. Unless it is an extremely hot day, only have the area that you are working on exposed. Nothing is worse than lying there trying to enjoy what should be a lovely, relaxing massage and instead being miserable with cold. Another way to prevent this is to use either a hot-water bottle, or a small heat pad.

Make sure that the room is warm beforehand – but don't try to give a long massage with an electric fan blowing, as it is noisy, dries out the air, and is exhausting for the person giving the massage.

Your comfort

When massaging you need to be comfortable. You often get oil on your clothes, and so you shouldn't wear anything that you would hate to ruin; so wear easy, preferably washable, loose-fitting clothes.

The way that you stand or kneel greatly influences the massage you give. If you are comfortable, the chances are that you will give a good massage. It is impossible to relax someone else if you yourself are twisted in an awkward position.

Try to use the weight of the whole of your body. If you are standing beside the table, have one leg slightly in front of the other, bend your knees and put the strength of your legs and back into the massage. Keep your back straight and lean the weight of the body forward, swaying your whole body and moving in rhythm with the massage movements. The same rule applies when kneeling. By using your body correctly, you are able to give a more even pressure throughout the massage and it prevents you from becoming exhausted.

To protect your own back, your posture is *very* important. Keep your back straight and bend from the hips and at the knees.

Hints

In this section I have tried to give you some hints about massage which are not just based on technique but which will give some 'spirit' to your massage. I am constantly surprised that today's massage training seems to lay all the emphasis on technique. The consequence is that the massage is clinical and soulless, which neither the giver nor the recipient really enjoy. Massage should be pleasurable.

Don't be afraid to be sensuous. After all, children are naturally very sensuous and 'touchy' and give extremely good massages. So if you have children and enjoy being massaged, train them quickly!

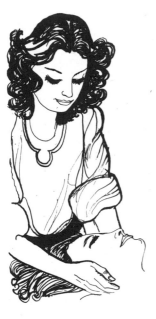

1. When massaging, don't worry if your movements become clumsy and you feel lost and cannot remember what to do next – everyone experiences this at first. It is simply a question of becoming familiar with the body. Even after years of experience I find that the first massage on a new person is never one of my best. I am getting the feel of their body and they are becoming used to, and therefore relaxing under, my hands. Just remember any form of touching feels good and will give pleasure and enjoyment.

When I massage, I try and imagine that it's me receiving the massage. Remember what feels good to *you*, because that will nearly always feel good to them. You can then *feel* how the movement should be. For instance, I love a rhythmic massage and so that is what I aim to give.

2. Glide your hands over the body, moulding your hands around the contours. Just let your hands flow easily, trying to make firm, reassuring strokes (not soft, hesitant ones) to convey a feeling of confidence.

3. Keep your hands in contact with the body throughout the massage, which maintains the flow of the massage. Suddenly stopping and starting again, and jerkily lifting your hands, breaks the rhythm.

4. Rhythm, rhythm, rhythm. It is the rhythmic flowing of one movement into another which makes massage so relaxing. Imagine that your hands are dancing over the body, the movements imperceptibly going into each other. Try massaging to music. You will find that your hands will instinctively keep time to the beat. Try all the different kinds of music possible, from classical to rock and reggae – each piece gives a different mood and consequently a different massage. The music will also help to make *you* relax into the massage.

5. When massaging, one way to make sure that your movements are going in the right direction is to think how you could make the body look neater and slimmer. In fact when I massage, I am mentally trying to mould the body into a more attractive form, 'Pull it in here, and up here,' etc. If you think in this way, your movements are bound to be correct. No one wants their body made wider or more flabby. What we want is to be firmer and neater and so your massage movements should be geared towards the moulding of the body into its perfect shape.

6. Make sure that the room is warm, the lights low, and that your friend is comfortable.

7. Try not to talk. Catch up on all the gossip some other time. Your massage will be much better if you concentrate on it. Pretend you're a professional and only talk a little, and in a low voice. See if you can send your friend to sleep.

Pressure

The pressure applied in massage varies from the very lightest touch to a firm heavy pressure.

Do not be scared to use pressure. Our bodies are really very strong and will not break; firm pressure feels good. You can apply pressure of 5 to 15 lbs with good effect – press down on your bathroom scales to see how much this is.

When I did training in *Shiatsu* (Japanese finger pressure massage, see page 138), my teacher used to shift all his weight onto his thumbs and bounce off the floor! Although the pressure was very heavy, he knew exactly what he was doing, so it didn't hurt. I am not recommending that you try this, but just want to show that you need not be scared of applying pressure, once you know how. Always check with your friend. You want to apply enough pressure to be effective but not to hurt – and this varies with each individual.

'The finger of a good rubber will descend upon an excited and painful nerve as gently as the dew on the grass and upon a torrid callosity as heavily as the hoof of an elephant.'
Beveridge, a Scots masseur,
1774–1839

In 500 BC a Greek physician thought that the pressure should be gentle at first, then greater in the middle and towards the end gentle again. This is still true today, and the way I would normally massage. In the early seventeenth century, Admiral Henry was of the opinion that heavy, violent massage was needed. The famous nineteenth-century masseur, Lucas Championnière, thought that massage should be slow and uniform – 'little more than a caress!' – an opinion which a German contemporary of his criticized: 'Massage which becomes painless ceases to be massage, only treatment by suggestion.'

Mennel (1880–1957), whose work is the foundation for most modern massage, believed that massage should be deep but not forcible, and that a delicate touch could do as much as a hard pressure. I agree with him. Your hands must be certain, but not hard enough to cause pain. If you hurt someone, their muscles tense up, thus destroying half the work you have done so far.

Rate, rhythm and pressure

In my opinion, these are the most important components of a good massage.

It is possible to do a whole massage using only the stroking movements. You can do the same movement over and over again and you make it feel different and enjoyable by simply changing the rate, rhythm and pressure.

In fact, I have frequently had professional, technically-good massages which I have enjoyed less than those of an unqualified friend because the former lacked these qualities.

So do not worry about it if you cannot manage to do some of the movements; with practice they will eventually come. Remember that with rhythm and pressure you can make the most simple massage feel good; so just relax and enjoy yourself.

Tension

When massaging, try and be aware of your friend's body. Is it soft and relaxed or taut and hard? If it feels stiff, tight or lumpy it can mean that tension has accumulated in those particular areas. So spend a little extra time massaging there.

Tickling
Ticklishness can often be caused by nervous tension and I find that if I slightly increase the pressure and persevere in that spot, it usually disappears. But if this doesn't work, just move on to another area.

Deep breathing
If your friend is tired and tense, help him (or her) to relax by breathing deeply. The best way to make someone more tense is to tell them to relax, so instead, when you start the massage, breathe slowly and deeply yourself. Stroke to the rhythm of your breathing. Very soon they will have picked up your rhythmic breathing, and will respond automatically.

Before you start
Read each movement through first. Do not try and learn too many different movements at a time. Until you get the feel of the body, just do the same strokes over and over again.

Try and persuade a friend to learn with you, it is ideal for couples. Practice on each other. To begin with, perhaps, the one being massaged could read the instructions aloud, as you actually work out the movements. This makes it much easier because then *both* of you can try and work out what I mean. Once you have mastered the movements then you can give your friend a really relaxing massage.

You will find that you learn as much by having a massage as you do by giving it. So do try and swop massages; you give the massage one day and receive it the next. Both are enjoyable. In fact, students of my massage courses tell me that they find doing the massage is just as relaxing as receiving it.

Before doing a massage check that your nails are not too long. Take off your rings and wash your hands in warm water.

One word of warning
Never massage anyone who is undergoing medical treatment, or who has a temperature, without your friend consulting a doctor first. Although you are trying to help, you might massage an inflamed nerve and that would only make things worse. *When in doubt do not massage.*

Anatomy
Although a knowledge of anatomy is useful, I don't think it is essential. You don't need to know the names of the muscles and bones – unless you want to impress other people!

What is useful, however, is to have an idea of the structure of the body; where the muscles are, whether they are large or small and what they do; where the bones are and what lies beneath them. You can work a lot of this out for yourself by simply looking at the body. For instance, bend your arm to see which muscles are working. But by looking at a chart, you will get a picture of the whole structure, and this will make you feel confident and at ease with the body.

In massage the main concern is with the muscles. There are over two hundred. They are like an intricate webbing, weaving together to make the fleshy covering of the body. Some are cord-like, some form thick masses and others are flat.

Most muscles are attached to two or more bones, and some are attached to the connective tissue adjoining other muscles. Movement is possible by groups of muscles working together, some relaxing, some contracting.

The diagrams are simply here to help you become familiar with the body – so that you can see where the bones, muscles and organs are located. Obviously you can apply more pressure to a large muscle than to a bone.

By keeping this picture in your mind you will soon become at ease and familiar with the body.

'Hard rubbing binds, soft rubbing loosens, much rubbing causes parts to waste; moderate rubbing makes them grow.'
Hippocrates, 460–380 B.C.

The back

> If you have just turned straight to this section and skipped my painfully worked out general blurb – please go back and read it. It is as important as the following description of technique.

I am going to start by showing you how to massage the back. There are several reasons for this. The first is that most people enjoy having their backs massaged, and that will give you confidence. Another is that as the back is a large area you have lots of space on which to practise all the different movements. And therefore a brief summary of the anatomy of the back is relevant here. Running down the centre of the back there is the spine. The spine consists of separate vertebrae from the base of the skull to the base of the lumbar. Of these, the cervicals are in the neck: in the mid-region are twelve thoracic vertebrae and in the lumbar region there are five vertebrae, the sacrum and the coccyx. The main muscles are easy to define: starting from the shoulders there are the trapezius, the deltoid, the sternocleidomastordens, the latissimus dorsi, the glutus maximus and glutus medius in the bottom.

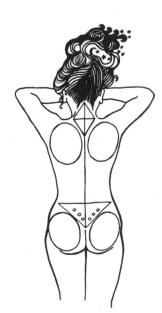

The spinal area in the back is the seat of the nervous system. Some spinal tension is necessary to maintain both rigidity and flexibility of the body, but too much causes discomfort, depression, fatigue and headaches. Back massage can release this excess tension giving a feeling of well-being and relaxation.

I always imagine the back to be made up of a series of triangles and circles. This is totally unscientific but I find that by keeping a picture like this in my mind, it is easier to flow from one movement to another.

Once you have mastered the massage of the back everything else will be easy for you.

Starting the back massage
First your friend must undress or at least take off the clothes covering the back. Men can keep on their trousers and simply undo their belt if they are shy – but if possible, you do want to be able to get down to the very base of the spine and buttocks.

Get your friend to lie face down; the arms can either be loosely bent with the hands at shoulder level, or lying relaxed at the sides – whichever is most comfortable. I have found that a rolled-up small towel or jersey placed under the forehead means that the head is straight down and it's still possible to breathe, but some people prefer having their head to one side.

If your friend cannot get comfortable, it could be that he or she needs support under the stomach or chest. If round-shouldered and the upper spine curves out, a large cushion is needed under the head and shoulders. But if he or she has a hollow back they will need a flattish pillow under the stomach. If your friend feels stiff after lying down on the stomach, it means support is needed somewhere. The main criterion is that whatever shape your friend is, you must ensure their complete comfort.

When you are sure both you and your friend are comfortable, put the oil on your hands and rub them together, thus warming your hands and the oil. Start by stroking it on.

When more oil is needed, as I've already mentioned, don't forget to pour the oil onto the back of one hand (don't stop moving it though, keep on stroking), and when you've replaced the bottle, with the other hand slide the oil off the back of the hand and onto the body. This might sound complicated but when you try it you will find that it is quite easy.

Now at last we get onto the actual movements.

1. *Stroking (sometimes known as effleurage)*
Always start by stroking. You use this stroke to apply the oil, to become aware of the area you are working on, for your friend to get used to your hands, and to generally warm, relax and soothe the whole area. This is both the easiest and most useful movement.

Start with your hands on the lower back with your thumbs on either side of the spine and the fingers pointing towards the head. Keeping the whole of your hands in contact slide them up the back; at the neck let your fingers mould around the top of the shoulders and then glide them down the sides of the back to the waist. Pull up at the waist, and in, as you return to the starting point.

This is a very rhythmic movement, firm when going up the back and gentle when gliding down. Remember my rhythym, rate and pressure, and in this movement apply the pressure down into the lower back, glide up on either side of the spine to the neck, pressure again as you move across the shoulder, glide down, and again pressure as you pull up at the waist on your return to the beginning.

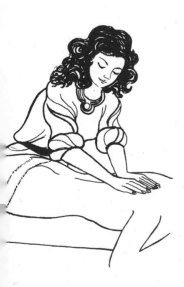

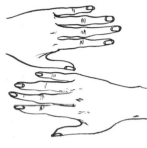

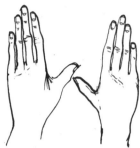

There are numerous variations to this stroking. Your hands can be facing each other with the fingers pointing towards the spine as you glide up. Or you can have one hand above the other with the thumb parallel to the little finger of the other hand.

The important thing to remember is to keep your hands firm but relaxed (this is rather difficult at first but with a little practise becomes easy), and let them mould around the contours of the body.

Do this main stroke about four or five times at the beginning of every massage. You will find it invaluable and can be used throughout your massage. Use it to soothe after you have done a stimulating movement; to help you glide from one movement into another; and most important, when you cannot think what to do next, do this while you decide. I have done a half-hour massage using only this movement: by varying the pressure and the speed it feels so different and is so relaxing, that it sometimes is all you need.

In some parts of the East relays of small boys were used to stroke the person being massaged. This gentle, light stroking is incredibly relaxing, and it has been used to induce a state of hypnosis.

Just remember – when in doubt – stroke!

2. *Friction*

Place the palms of your hands on the back and keeping them tense, rub them energetically backwards and forwards in short swift movements – just as you might do when trying to warm someone up. For once your hands do not mould around the body, but rub over the surface. This, exactly as its name implies, creates friction. It is especially useful if it is cold as it will warm both of you up! It's rather tiring, so don't do too much.

Follow by doing a few large stroking movements to soothe and calm the back. In fact, whenever you do a hard, fast movement, always follow with large soothing strokes.

3. *Kneading*

Don't be put off this movement by the rather complicated description – it sounds much more difficult than it is. Imagine that you are kneading bread and then it will come easily. This 'bread kneading' is a deep, stimulating movement. It is used on the underlying muscles and fatty areas, it stretches shortened muscles and tissue, and helps to relax hard, contracted muscles. It also greatly improves the circulation.

Make a kneading circular movement, using the heel of the hand and the fingers, compressing the flesh by repeatedly grasping and releasing it with alternate hands. Get a rhythm going, with one hand grasping, compressing and then releasing, and then the next – a rolling, flowing movement.

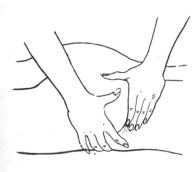

The hands can either work by pressing in the same direction, or imagine that you are wringing out a towel and try that on the fatty, hip area – or anywhere you can pick up a handful of flesh. Be careful not to pinch with the fingers. Try and keep the hands relaxed and the whole palm in contact with the contours of the body. (You can easily practise this movement on your own thighs.)

Start on the buttocks and hips, up the side of the body to the shoulders and down the other side. At the shoulders do the same movement, but instead of using the whole hand (it is too big and feels awkward) use your thumbs and the two middle fingers. When you have done several rows of kneading all around the fleshy area on either side of the neck, go down the side of the back nearest you to the base of the spine. And repeat.

It is easy doing this on the side away from you, but it can be slightly more difficult doing the side nearest you. You have to pull up with the thumbs, or you can move to the other side of the body, but this tends to break the continuity of the massage. Instead, I cheat slightly by twisting my body around as though I had moved. Be careful not to be uncomfortable yourself, though.

4. *Circular stroking*

This is virtually the same movement as the initial stroking, but instead of stroking up the sides of the spine simultaneously, you do a sweeping circular movement, one hand following the other. Start with the hands on either side of the spine and, with alternate hands, do a large circular movement up the side of the spine, and as you glide one hand back, the other hand goes up. A very easy movement to do.

This can also be done by making small circles on either side of the body, simultaneously, going up towards the shoulder and gliding back down the sides into the waist and up to the base of the spine. Again, when in doubt as to what to do, use this invaluable stroke.

5. *Pressures up the spine and neck*

(a)   This consists of making small circular movements up either side of the spine. You don't work on the spine itself, but in the furrows on either side. Beside the spine there are ridges of muscle which are frequently tense and hard. You can do these circular pressures with either your thumbs or your middle fingertips. Try both ways and see which you find the easiest.

Make a deep circular movement, then relax the pressure and glide up about half an inch. Press, circle, relax, glide; press, circle, relax, glide. This movement is very easy to do rhythmically and you can go either fast or slow.

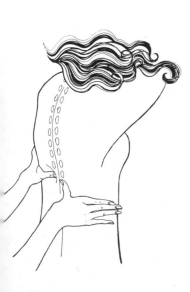

Work all the way up from the base of the spine to the top of the neck. Try to move the muscles away from the spine, as with this movement you are trying to relax and ease the tautness. Do pressures all around the triangle at the base of the neck (refer to the diagram). Having covered that, work up the neck to the hairline. Work all around the hairline and then glide the hands down to the base of the spine to start again. Repeat the process several times.

As well as muscles, there are spinal nerves running along on either side of the spine like a motorway going from the brain to the rest of the body, and this is why having this area massaged is so tremendously relaxing.

(b)   Again starting at the base of the back. With your fingers pointing

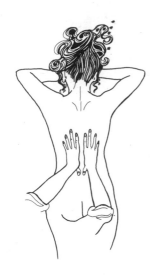

towards the head and the thumbs towards the bottom on either side of the spine, simply press the thumbs down and then glide up; press, glide; press, glide. This is a rhythmic but *bouncy* movement. The fingers are only there to lead you and all the pressure is in the thumbs. It is very easy to do and feels wonderful. Work up the spine a couple of times, gliding back down to start again.

6. *Pressures around the shoulders*

Staying at the top of the back do a large circular stroking around the shoulders. Rest one hand across the top of the other and press down on the heel of the hand and then make a deep, circular movement. Make several pressures in one area, then relax the hand and glide on, without losing contact, to the next area. Keep the lower hand relaxed and in full contact with the skin. Remember the hand is not moving the skin surface, but the underlying muscle. Do these pressures all over the shoulder area. Pressure should be firm, but not so heavy as to hurt the underlying tissue.

7. *Circling the shoulder blade*

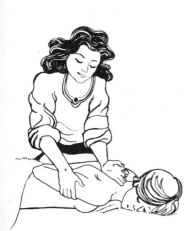

At first this might be a rather awkward movement to do, especially if you are working on the floor. Bend your friend's right arm and rest the back of the hand on the small of the back so that the shoulder blade protrudes. Start by lifting the point of the shoulder with your right hand; simultaneously run your left hand under the shoulder blade. The right hand glides down to the elbow, followed by the left hand. Return the right hand to the shoulder as the left hand completes a full circle from the elbow to under the shoulder blade. The pressure of the left hand is firm under the shoulder blade and around the shoulder, but necessarily lighter to flow from the elbow onto the back. The feeling is of a continuous double circle.

Do this three times on the right side and then replace the hand and do the same stroke on the other side. This time the left hand lifts the shoulder and the right hand does the complete circle.

You will probably find one side easier to do than the other, but persevere, and with a little practice it will soon become smooth and easy.

This is a very useful stroke as those large trapezius muscles are used a great deal. There is often a lot of tension in this area, and by lifting the shoulder you can work on it. By pulling up at the shoulder, it also slightly stretches the muscles of the chest.

Now do the first stroking movements over the whole back to make it all feel connected again.

8. *Bottom massage*

Some people are rather embarrassed about massaging the bottom; but if you can overcome this, it is incredibly relaxing. Massage will improve the circulation and relieve tension. We always tend to forget that this part of the body is alive – it's sat on and forgotten.

(a) Stroke the whole area with alternate circles. Starting with the hands on each buttock, slide the hands to the sides of the hips and complete the circle by pulling firmly in and back to the top of the buttocks.

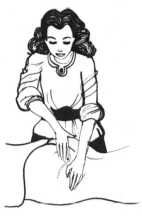

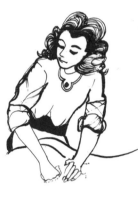

One can also work on one buttock at a time with both hands, using a circular movement similar to that which you used on the shoulder.

(b)   Just below the waist on either side of the spine there are three sets of pressure points which are worth finding because pressure here is so relaxing. Some people make life easy by having dimples where the top pressure points are, but if your friend doesn't, you can find them by pulling the buttocks up at the side, which usually makes these small indents visible. Place the thumbs on these indents with the fingers relaxed at the side of the body for balance. Press firmly and relax; press and relax. Then glide down to the centre of each side of the triangle, press and relax; press and relax. Finally glide down to the last one right at the base of the coccyx, press and relax; press and relax (see diagram).

Due to the fact that nearly everyone has terrible posture, there is usually a lot of tension in the lower back, so massage in this area is always particularly relaxing and enjoyable. It is especially effective in relieving the aching back that some women experience during menstruation.

(c)   There is a large pressure point in the middle of each buttock which can sometimes be seen as a light indentation. With relaxed fists simultaneously make a large circular movement in these hollows, and then stroke the whole area. This is a strong movement which seems to suit men particularly. Stroke the whole back again before the next movement.

9.   *Caterpillar walking*

Years ago a Japanese woman taught me how to walk up and down the back. This feels wonderful but does not usually fit easily into a normal massage and so I invented this caterpillar walk to get the same effect.

This is a rocking, climbing movement and the only one where you actually work on the spine itself. Start with your right hand at the base of the spine, the middle of the palm resting on the bone and your fingers on either side of the spine, facing towards the head. Put your left hand across the fingers of your right hand.

Press down on the fingers of your right hand as you lift up the heel of this hand, rolling the palm forward to place it as close to your fingers as possible. Then lift up the fingers, move them forward until your palm is flat, and press down.

It's rather difficult to describe this movement, but it feels so good, it's worth trying it. Your hand caterpillars up the spine, and down again. It is a bouncy, rocking movement with the pressure applied by the fingers – press, lift, down; press, lift, down. Finish up at the shoulder area for the next movement.

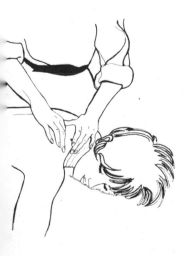

10.   *Piano playing*

If you play the piano, you will find this movement easy; imagine you are pressing down hard on the key-board, the fingers drumming on the fleshy area on either side of the neck. A lot of people suffer from fibrositis and tension in this area and this is a terrific movement for easing their stiffness. A lovely bouncy movement, but slightly tiring to do for long.

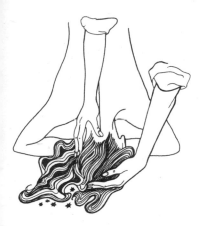

11. *Pressures on the neck*

With *one* hand do circular pressures up the neck, using the thumb and fingers on either side of the neck. Rest your other hand on your friend's head, which makes the movement more controlled and easier for you, and it's reassuring for them. The head can either be facing down or resting on one side – or, better still, do a little in both positions. Massage all around the base of the skull, slowly moving out to the ears, and then back to the centre again. Press gently with the thumb in the hollow at the top of the spine. Continue doing circular pressures up into the hair at the top of the head.

Most people accumulate a lot of tension in the neck, and massage will relieve it.

> **A word of warning**
> When massaging the neck be careful *not* to apply heavy pressure to the carotid artery – this would stop the blood flowing to the brain and can cause dizziness and blackouts.

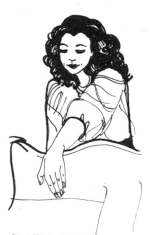

12. *Criss-crossing*

Start with your hands relaxed, both facing away from you on either side of the back and slide them back and forth across the body. Criss-crossing the hands and squeezing the body, pulling up at the sides and gliding over the centre. Do this over the entire back and the buttocks. Try varying the speed and the depth of the movement for different effects. You can also do this movement up and down the back; pulling down at the top of the back, pressing down into the waist and gliding over the middle. This is another very easy movement. If you are standing to do your massage, bend your knees as you pull across so that you get an easy rhythmic movement.

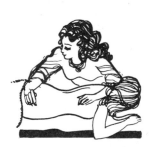

13. *Stretching the back*

Place your forearms across the middle of the back. Pressing down hard, slowly slide your arms apart, until one has reached the base of the skull and the other the buttocks. Hold the pressure there for a second then relax the arms and softly and smoothly return to the beginning. Repeat. Do this centred on the spine itself and then centred on either side of the back. This gives a fantastic stretching sensation and makes one feel taller.

14. *Slapping, percussion movements*

These consist of a series of soft, brisk blows, applied with alternate hands. The wrists are kept very flexible so that the movement is light, springy and stimulating. Although traditionally these movements are done at the end of the massage, they are apt to wake one up rather brutally, which seems a shame when you have spent all that time making your friend sleepy and relaxed. So experiment and see where you like to use them in your massage. (The Zen Buddhists use a sharp slap on the shoulder muscle as they believe it has a stimulating effect on a wandering mind!)

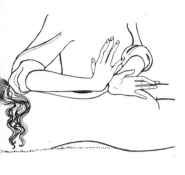

(a)   *Hacking* is done with the side of the hands, with relaxed fingers and wrists. When you are doing it correctly you can hear the sound of your fingers knocking together. Use this on the buttocks, up the side of the body and over the shoulders, but never on bony areas.

To make sure that you don't hurt your friend practise it on the side of a table – if that doesn't hurt you, then it won't hurt your friend.

(b)   *Clapping* is nearly the same movement but this time your relaxed, slightly cupped hands should drop loosely onto the body and immediately spring off again. This makes a very impressive hollow clapping sound. It is the movement that you always see in James Bond films!

(c)   *Pummelling* used to be practised by travellers in the East, and I think this is something we ought to copy. Office workers tend to develop large behinds and thighs, and if we pummelled ourselves this would increase the circulation, and stimulate the whole area.

This time you have loosely clenched hands and pummel with the ulna side of the hand (thumbs up and little fingers down).

Personally this is the only percussion movement that I like and I use it all over the back. Do it quite gently with very relaxed wrists and hands as if you were playing the maraccas. It's a very rhythmic movement, and you can vary the speed for different effects. If done quite slowly it is very relaxing and can be used at the end of the massage.

You can also do these vigorous movements near the beginning of a massage as they release tension and are surprisingly enjoyable.

15.   *Stroking down the spine*
This is a lovely relaxing movement. Place the whole hand at the base of the neck, and slowly, but firmly, stroke down the back; as you reach the base of the spine follow with the other hand. Smoothly lift the first hand off the back and replace it at the top ready to follow the other hand, so that you are always in contact with the back. This is a continuous, extremely relaxing and soothing movement. Start with quite a fast, firm movement, and gradually get slower and slower, and softer and softer.

It is as lovely to do as it is to receive; inducing sleep in both the person being massaged and the masseur – in fact when I'm giving my massage courses, my students become completely relaxed and sleepy just by watching.

16.   *Feather touch*
This is a continuation of the last movement. Using the finger tips of both hands and barely touching the skin, stroke down the back. At the base of the back gently lift the hands off and flick them before returning to the beginning again. Gently shake your hands as if you are shaking off water between the large strokes. This dispels any electricity that gathers in the hands. Repeat several times.

17.   *The final touch*
Lay your relaxed, slightly cupped hands next to each other at the base of the spine. Just hold them there and you will be amazed to find that

the area under your hands will start to feel warm. Give a gentle slow pressure, relax the hands and *slowly* lift them off the body.

Pull a towel up to cover the back and hopefully you will have a very relaxed friend lying there half asleep.

Once you have mastered the massage of the back, you will find the rest of the body incredibly easy.

Quick check list for your back massage

1.	Stroking	10.	Piano playing
2.	Friction	11.	Pressures on the neck
3.	Kneading	12.	Criss-crossing
4.	Circular stroking	13.	Stretching the back
5.	Pressures up spine and neck	14.	Slapping movements
6.	Pressures around shoulders	15.	Stroking down the spine
7.	Circling the shoulder blade	16.	Feather touch
8.	Bottom massage	17.	The final touch
9.	Caterpillar walking		

You have now done all the basic movements of massage: stroking, kneading, pressures and slapping. And it is very easy to adapt all these movements to the different parts of the body. It is simply a question of adapting the movements to fit the area.

When learning massage, I think the leg is the next area to tackle, one of the reasons being that it is the next largest, and therefore easiest, area to learn on. Another is that our legs get extremely tired and tense from walking or standing all day, and it is a great relief to have them massaged.

The thighs need massage because so many suffer from slightly thick thighs which can be improved by a bit of pummelling to increase their circulation and tone up the muscles.

The calves can get very tense, especially if you're on your feet all day. And for us city dwellers the hard pavements are as bad for us as they are for the horses in this childish rhyme: 'It's not the 'opping over 'edges that 'arms the 'orses 'ooves, but the 'ammer, 'ammer, 'ammer on the 'ard 'igh road!'

And as for the feet, it is so important to massage them that I have given them a special section. I always start a leg massage by massaging the foot as this has the most relaxing effect on nearly everyone. And that makes it easier for you, and more enjoyable for your friend.

The foot

I think that the foot is one of the three areas that most benefit from massage, the other two being the back and the head. Although our poor feet are the hardest working part of the body we tend to cram them into our shoes and forget them – they get nothing like the attention they deserve. Leonardo da Vinci referred to the foot as 'the greatest engineering device in the world'. We have twenty-eight separate bones in each foot and an intricate webbing of muscles. There are thousands of nerve endings in the sole of the foot and by massaging these it is thought that we can relax or stimulate the rest of the body as well. In zone therapy and reflexology the foot is thought of as a map of the body, and illness can be treated by massaging it (see page 143). But for our purpose now it is enough to know that by massaging the feet, you can make your friend feel marvellously relaxed.

So let's begin the actual massage, with your friend lying face up. Just as in the back, you start by stroking, which is the best way of applying the oil, and warming and relaxing the whole leg.

Stand or kneel to the side of your friend's calf facing the head. Pour oil into the palms of your hands, rub your hands together to warm them and then start.

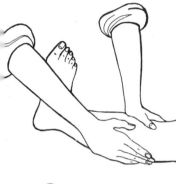

1. *Stroking the whole leg*
(a)   Grasp the ankle with both hands and then stroke up the sides of the leg. Apply pressure as you go up and then glide down, moulding your relaxed hands around the contours of the leg. Do this about four times.

(b)   Now with your hands across the leg, starting at the ankle, stroke firmly up the front of the calf to the top of the thigh and glide gently down the sides, continuing right down to the toes. Repeat four times.

After the preliminary stroking of the whole leg, we do the foot massage.

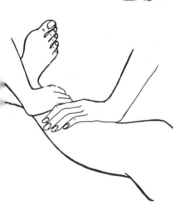

2. *Stroking the foot*
(a)   Stroke down the top of the foot from the toes to the ankles with both hands and glide back with one hand on either side of the foot. Repeat rhythmically and firmly, several times. A lot of people suffer from bad circulation and consequently have cold feet. This firm stroking stimulates the circulation and warms them up.

(b)   Clasp the toes between your palms and make a large circular movement simultaneously on the top of and the sole of the foot. This movement, as with all stroking, can be used at any time throughout your massage. When in doubt – stroke!

3. *Circling*
(a)   Start with crossed thumbs at the base of the toes and with your fingers held lightly under the foot. Make a firm stroke down the front of the foot and glide around and back to the starting position. An easy relaxed circular movement, concentrating on the area below the toes.

(b)   Circling the ankles, use your two middle fingers to make small rotaries all around the bone, working on both sides at once. Be thorough and firm. Massage all around the ankle is extremely soothing. Nagging back-ache caused by period pains can be alleviated by simply massaging here.

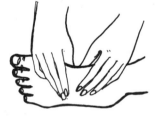

(c)   Move back to the toes. Support the foot with one hand and work with the other. With your thumb and finger start working on the little toe. Holding it firmly, stroke the top and bottom surfaces, and then apply rotary pressures on each side. Stroke down then rotate, two circles one way and two the other and then pull it. Repeat once. Rotaries, stroke, rotate and pull. Continue along the toes until you reach the big toe (I find it easiest if I change hands now) where you repeat three times. Do these toe rotaries unhurriedly and smoothly. End by grasping all the toes together and flexing them back and forth.

(d)   Now move down to the crevices that you can see between the tendons of the foot. Support the foot at a right angle to the leg as this makes the furrows more visible and stretches the achilles tendon. With the thumb do circular pressures down the foot from the toes to the ankles. As you work down these furrows with one hand, support the foot with the other. Again you will find that it is easier if you change your hands around half-way through.

4.   *Pressures*

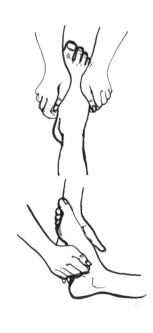

(a)   An Oriental client was taught this movement by her father, a famous politician, whose feet she used to massage daily to release tension. Hold the foot, with your thumbs behind the toes and your fingers resting across them. With your thumbs, press hard into the sole of the foot. Press hard, hold the pressure and release. Move down a little and repeat the pressure, work in a straight line down the centre of the foot to the heel. Glide back to the beginning and repeat.

(b)   With your fingers resting on the front of the foot apply pressure to the instep with your thumbs. Make a jerky scissor-like movement across the top of the foot with the fingers whilst pressing up with the thumbs. Scissor up and down the whole foot. It feels terrific, relieves tension and when done at the top of the foot separates the toes.

(c)   This is a continuation of the last movement but this time you stretch the foot by squeezing it down and pulling it up. Press down with the fingers on top of the foot while pushing up with the thumbs, squeezing the foot into itself. Then reverse the process and stretch the foot by pulling up with the thumbs and fingers. Easy to do, and it feels wonderful. Squeeze and stretch, squeeze and stretch.

(d)   Support the top of the foot with one hand and make a fist with the other. Move your knuckles loosely but firmly in circles all around the sole of the foot.

(e)   This is a large circular pressure down into the instep. Really mould the rounded heel of the hand into the hollow of the instep. Again this is very easy to do, and very soothing to the person being massaged.

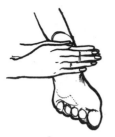

5. *Slapping the foot*
Use the hacking movement that we did on the back, on the sole of the foot, and even with discretion on the bony top. This feels surprisingly good.

6. *Rotating the foot*
With one hand at the ankle for support and the other holding the ball of the foot slowly rotate it in a large circle three times one way and then the other. It is amazing how stiff peoples' ankles can be, and so go gently.

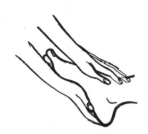

7. *Clasping the foot*
As a final touch to the foot massage, stroke the whole foot as you did at the beginning and then clasp the foot between your palms. Firmly but gently pull it towards you. Relax and repeat a couple of times gradually becoming gentler and gentler.

People are very funny about their feet; they either love having them massaged or they feel very embarrassed and tense about it. Some people complain of having ticklish feet, but this will disappear with a few firm movements. Anyhow, try experimenting and see.

The leg

Now that you have finished the foot massage you move on up to the calf and thigh. Your friend should still be lying face up.

The calf
1. *Stroking*
With the palms of your hands on either side of the ankle, stroke firmly up the side of the calf to the knee, and return by gliding the hands down the front of the calf. I find it easiest if I use the heel of my hand to apply the pressure when going up, as this gives a lot of strength with very little effort.

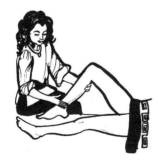

2. *Pressures up the side of the shin*
Hold the ankle loosely with one hand, and with the fingers of the other hand under the leg and the thumb by the side of the shin bone, do circular pressures with the thumb up one side of the bone to the knee and glide back down. Repeat twice, then change hands and do the same on other side of the bone.

3. *Alternate strokes up the calf*
Lift the leg at the knee with the foot resting on the ground. Support the leg and keep it in place by sitting next to it.

With alternate hands stroke up the calf, pulling the muscle up and out to the side, gliding down between the strokes. This is an easy, large, circular, rhythmic movement.

4. *Chinese torture*
I nearly did not include this movement because I don't particularly like it (and it's so difficult to explain), but at a recent massage course

for men they voted it the most effective and enjoyable leg movement. Their enthusiasm spurred me into using it again and I have found everyone loves it. It is especially good on men and athletes who have tight calf muscles.

With the leg in the same position as for the previous movement, place your hands around the ankle, fingers underneath and thumbs across the top. Keeping the whole hand in contact with the leg, press the fingers firmly down around, the hands moving towards each other and criss-crossing around the calf (a movement reminiscent of the Chinese Torture we inflicted on each other at school). Criss-cross across the calf up to the knee and back. Repeat three times and then, supporting the leg at the knee and ankle; straighten and relax the leg down, ready for the next movement.

The knee
You might not think it was particularly pleasurable and relaxing to have your knees massaged – but it is. Try these three movements and see for yourself. It's really lovely.

1. *Circling around the knee with the thumbs*
Starting with crossed thumbs below the knee-cap, move both thumbs up around the sides of the knee, uncross them at the top of the knee and bring them down the other sides to the beginning again. This sounds complicated, but it isn't when you try it. Repeat several times.

2. *Circling the knee with the hand*
The same movement at the last one, but this time circle the knee with the whole hand.

3. *Rotaries around the knee*
Slide your fingers under the knee and do gentle rotary pressures there using your finger tips. There is a very large pressure point here and so this easy movement is incredibly soothing and relaxing. *Another* one of my favourites!

The thigh
Although massaging the thighs obviously does have a soothing, relaxing quality I find its main use is in improving the shape. All these movements increase the circulation and so are particularly beneficial to anyone who suffers from large thighs, lumps, bumps and cellulite (see page 117).

Women frequently complain of thick thighs, and I have numerous clients on whom I spend a whole hour massaging only their thighs, especially just before the summer holidays when some have massage every single day. The massage improves the muscle tone and generally greatly improves their appearance. If you massage your *own* thighs conscientiously you will see a marked improvement.

1. *Stroking*
With the palms of your hands on either side of the knee, stroke firmly

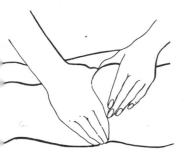

up the side of the thigh and return by gliding the hands down the front. Applying the pressure with the heels of your hands when you go up, and releasing it when you gently slide back.

2. *Kneading and wringing*
This is an ideal place to practise your 'bread-kneading' (see page 90), as most of us have a little extra fat here. From the knee, work up the outside of the thigh, pushing the flesh up towards the centre, then in the middle of the thigh and then on the inside. In other words work all over the thigh. For variety, try putting an extra twist into your kneading, as though you were wringing out a towel.

3. *Rolling up the thigh*
Start with your hands just above the knee, on either side of the thigh. Pressing with the heel and palm of the hand, roll the muscle against the bone. With the hands circling alternately, move up the thigh and glide down. This rolling movement always reminds me of the mechanism of the old steam train wheels. Repeat several times.

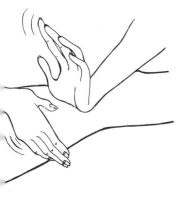

4. *Alternate stroking*
With alternate hands stroke firmly up the thigh with large circular movements. As with all massage on the thigh, the pressure is on the upward stroke.

5. *Hacking and pummelling*
Hack and pummel on the outer thigh. Remember that this is a bouncy, upward movement which should stimulate but not hurt. If your friend suffers from broken veins, avoid them.

6. *Stroking the whole leg*
Stroke the whole leg from the ankle to the thigh. Start with firm rhythmic strokes and get steadily slower and gentler until you are barely touching the skin – the feather touch, which is so soothing and sleep inducing.

7. *The final touch*
On the last stroke clasp the foot between the palms of your hands, press firmly and then very steadily pull the whole leg towards you, slowly release the pressure and gradually slide your hands away.

You have now completed the leg massage. Move over and massage the other leg, otherwise your poor friend will feel lopsided.

'The physician must be experienced in many things but assuredly also in rubbing. For rubbing can bind a joint that is too loose and loosen a joint that is too rigid.'

Hippocrates, 460–380 BC

Quick check list for the leg and foot massages

The foot

The foot
1. Stroking the whole leg
2. Stroking the foot
3. Circling
4. Pressures
5. Slapping the foot
6. Rotating the foot
7. Clasping the foot

The knee
1. Circling around the knee with the thumbs
2. Circling the knee with the hand
3. Rotaries around the knee

The thigh
1. Stroking
2. Kneading and wringing
3. Rolling up the thigh

The leg

The calf
1. Stroking
2. Pressures up the side of the shin
3. Alternate strokes up the calf
4. Chinese torture

4. Alternate stroking
5. Hacking and pummelling
6. Stroking the whole leg
7. The final touch

The stomach

It is surprisingly relaxing to have your stomach massaged. If you have a stomach ache, simple stroking will relieve it, and it is also calming for indigestion and period pains. Tummy massage is particularly good if you are on a diet or you've just had a baby, as it helps tone up the muscles, and makes you more aware of the area.

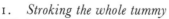

1. *Stroking the whole tummy*
With the hands on the stomach, pointing towards the face, stroke up the ribs, open out the hands and glide down the sides to the beginning. Repeat this easy rhythmic movement several times.

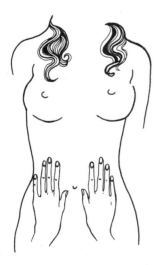

2. *Stroking around the lower abdomen*
This is a circular stroking over the colon, which lies in a curve from hip to hip in the lower part of the stomach. Place one hand on each hip bone and while your left hand circles clockwise and makes the top half of a circle, simultaneously your right hand completes the bottom half. The hands follow each other so it feels like a continuous flowing movement, rather like rubbing one's tummy when one has eaten too much. A soothing movement.

3. *Kneading on the sides*

Work around the waist and up the sides. Using the whole hand pick up and squeeze the flesh. Work with alternate hands (facing each other), just as though you are kneading bread. If your friend is trying to reduce, this is the movement to use as it is stimulating. This is easy on the hips and waist but may be difficult over the ribs as there tends to be less flesh there, in which case just open the hand out more and be careful not to pinch. Use the thumb and middle fingers to do small kneading movements all over the stomach and rib cage. Work thoroughly over the entire area.

4. *Pressures on the colon*

With the palm of the hand make circular pressures in a clockwise direction around the colon. For a steady controlled pressure, place one hand on top of the other and keep your hands relaxed. Press down, rotate, relax and glide half a hand's width along. Press, rotate, relax, glide. I find that if I let my fingers trail between the pressures it makes the movement smoother and thus more soothing.

5. *Criss-crossing the tummy*

This is exactly the same movement as we used on the back. Start with your hands facing away from you on either side of the abdomen, and slide them back and forth across the body. Criss-crossing across the stomach, pulling up at the sides and gliding over the centre. Do it at least six times.

6. *Lifting the back*

At the waist slide your hands, one on either side, beneath your friend's back to the spine. With your fingers make a few circular rotaries on either side of the spine and then gently lift up the back, hold for a second, and smoothly and firmly pull your hands back around to the stomach again. When your hands are there, press gently down. Repeat the whole movement several times. This is another of my favourite movements, as it's such a lovely comforting feeling to be pulled up like this. A word of warning though. It could be a bit of a strain on your own back so make sure that you are comfortable and use the strength of your body to lift correctly.

7. *Deep stroking up the abdomen*

With your hands next to each other, the heels at the base of the abdomen and the fingers pointing towards the face, gently press them down, and maintaining the same strong pressure push them infinitely slowly up the stomach to the rib cage, where you release the pressure and glide your hands around the waist and back to the stomach. Repeat several times. This is a very long, deep, steady stroke which takes me about 45 seconds to complete – and that is much longer than you'd think.

I learnt this movement in India when the local flower-seller gave me a massage. She told me that they use it to help the stomach back into its proper place after childbirth. Whether you are in need of that or not, it is a lovely movement, so do try it. It's very easy to do and feels terrific.

8. *Stroking the whole stomach*
Rhythmically stroke the whole stomach with the pressure becoming softer and softer. End by doing the feather touch down the stomach — just trail your fingers as lightly as possible down the centre.

9. *The final touch*
Place the palms of your hands, slightly cupped, with the fingers overlapping across the middle of the stomach (over the tummy button). Hold them there for a few seconds, press down gently and then gradually release the pressure. Repeat twice. This simple pressure has the most incredibly relaxing effect and is the perfect end to your tummy massage.

Quick check list for your stomach massage

		5.	Criss-crossing the tummy
1.	Stroking the whole tummy	6.	Lifting the back
2.	Stroking lower abdomen	7.	Deep stroking up the abdomen
3.	Kneading on the sides	8.	Stroking the whole stomach
4.	Pressures on the colon	9.	The final touch

The chest

I only do a few movements on the chest. One is easy to do as a continuation of the tummy massage, and I usually incorporate the other two into my face and head massages.

1. *Stroking up the chest*
Place your hands on the abdomen and slide them up over the chest towards the neck. Open out the hands with the thumbs on the collar bone and your fingers at the back of the neck. Press down and knead and squeeze this area, then slide your hands out to the shoulders. Gently press them down and then glide back to the waist. Repeat this relaxing stroking movement several times.

The following movements I do from behind the head.

2. *Stroking down the chest*
Place the palms of your hands at the base of the neck on the collar bone, your fingers making a V. Slide them down the chest to the breast, pull them out to the shoulders and press them down. Then swivel the hands around the shoulder points so that your palms cup them and glide up the neck. Slowly and gently pull the head towards you, then glide your hands back to the front. Repeat this relaxing movement several times.

3. *Knuckling the chest*
Using your knuckles make small circular 'knuckling' movements all

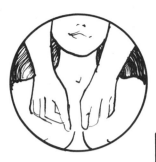

over the chest. Men seem to like this particularly. Some people accumulate their tension in the chest, and this movement relaxes it.

Finish by stroking the whole area again. As I have said before, stroking always feels good and you can make it feel different by simply varying the speed and pressure.

Quick check list for your chest massage

1. Stroking up the chest
2. Stroking down the chest
3. Knuckling the chest

The arm and hand

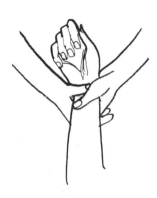

There are several good reasons for massaging the arm and hand. Massage relieves the tension that can accumulate in the arms either through carrying heavy weights or over-use – typists, tennis players, gardeners and writers frequently suffer from stiff arms. Sometimes you don't even realize that the muscles are taut until they are massaged and then with all the tension alleviated, they feel completely different.

Massage helps increase the circulation, and so it is useful if anyone suffers from excessively cold hands, or that red, blotchy, goose-pimply skin on the upper arms. Older people tend to suffer from stiff hands and swollen joints, and although one must never massage an inflamed area, light massage can be very soothing, and can alleviate the stiffness.

The massage of the arm and hand is virtually the same as that for the leg and foot and so you should find that it presents no new difficulties.

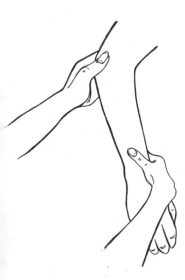

The hand

1. *Stroking the whole arm*
Start with your hands laid across the wrist, one hand above the other, with the thumb parallel to the little finger of the other hand. Stroke firmly up to the shoulder, the hands moulded across the arm, and glide gently down the sides. With this initial stroking you apply the oil, improve the circulation and relax the arm before going on to massage the hand.

2. *Stroking the hand*
Start with your fingers supporting the palms and with your thumbs crossed on the knuckles. Make firm strokes down towards the wrist and relax the pressure to circle back.

3. *Massaging the fingers*
Use one of your hands as a support and massage with the other. With

your thumb and index finger, grasp the little finger and apply circular pressures around the knuckles, then work on all the joints up to the tip. Glide back to the knuckles and apply the same circular pressures on either side of the finger. Then grasp the finger firmly at the middle joint and rotate the finger, first one way and then the other. Make a large definite circle. End by grasping the finger and giving it a long steady pull towards you. You can feel the knuckle separating and in some people this produces a cracking sound. Then move onto the next finger, ending with the thumb.

4.   *Pressures between the tendons*
Support the palm of the hand with the fingers of your hands and use your thumbs to do circular pressures into the furrows between the tendons. Work down each of these crevices to the wrist. Finish with a rhythmic, firm, stroking movement in the furrows from the knuckles to the wrist.

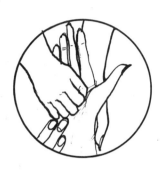

5.   *Kneading the palm*
Turn your friend's hand over and hold it palm up. With the heel of your other hand, knead the palm. Now make a fist with your hand and move your knuckles in small circles all over the palm. Then using your thumb, make deep circular pressures around the palm – especially in the centre, where there is a pressure point and if it is stimulated it should help to increase your energy.

6.   *Stretching and squeezing the hand*
Enclose the hand, palm down, with your thumbs on top and your fingers underneath. Squeeze the hand tightly, like a crunching handshake, and stretch it out by pulling up the sides. This is an extremely useful, easy movement which relaxes the whole hand.

7.   *Stroking the whole hand*
To end the hand massage stroke the whole hand several times.

The arm
1.   *Alternate stroking on the inside of the forearm*
Lift up your friend's forearm, leaving the elbow on the floor or table. Clasp your hands around the wrist with the thumbs on the inside. Press down with your thumbs, making large firm alternate strokes down to the elbow, with one thumb following the other. The thumbs may describe a circle, or a simple up-down stroke.

2.   *Rotary pressures up the arm*
Loosely support the wrist with the palm of the hand, and with the thumb of the other hand, do the rotaries. Start at the wrist and do three lines of rotary pressures up the forearm to the elbow. One line on either side of the arm and one in the middle.

3.   *Circling the elbow*
Still supporting the wrist with one hand, bend the elbow slightly and using your fingers and thumb do rotary pressures all around the elbows, working in all the little crevices. Then with the whole of your hand circle around the elbow. Beside feeling good, the elbow skin is nearly

always dry and horny and will soak up the oil.

4. *Stroking the upper arm*

Enclosing the arm with both your hands, stroke up from the elbow to the shoulder. As usual, a firm rhythmic stroking.

5. *Kneading the upper arm*

Do the bread-kneading which you used on the upper thigh. Knead all over the upper arm either with your hands together or try it with one hand on each side of the arm. This movement is especially good for improving bad circulation.

6. *Rolling up the arm*

Starting from the elbow, with one hand on either side of the arm, apply firm pressure and roll the muscle against the bone with rhythmic alternate circles. Work from the elbow up to the shoulder, glide down and repeat.

7. *Stroking the whole arm*

Stroke the upper arm a couple of times and then stroke the whole arm, fast at first and getting steadily slower and gentler. Finish by stroking with your fingertips hardly touching the skin, a light feather touch. End up at the hand for the last movement.

8. *The final touch*

Clasp the hand between your palms and apply a firm pressure, and then very steadily pull the whole arm gently towards you. The movement shouldn't pull the shoulder towards you, but just stretches out the arm. Still holding the hand allow the arm to relax back. Apply one last pressure to the hand and then relax the pressure and gradually slide your hands away.

It is always a good idea to make the ending of any part of your massage feel smooth and definite, otherwise it feels most disconcerting when one is being massaged and it suddenly, and abruptly comes to an end. These final movements are worth practising, as it is this which will make your massage feel professional.

Now you have finished one arm and so you should move over to massage the other.

Quick check list for the arm and hand massage

The hand

1. Stroking the whole arm
2. Stroking the hand
3. Massaging the fingers
4. Pressures between the tendons.
5. Kneading the palm
6. Stretching the hand
7. Stroking the whole hand

The arm

1. Alternate stroking on forearm
2. Rotary pressures up the arm
3. Circling the elbow
4. Stroking the upper arm
5. Kneading the upper arm
6. Rolling up the arm
7. Stroking the whole arm
8. The final touch

The face and head

Why does one massage the face and head?

Primarily because it feels so wonderful. A tremendous amount of tension accumulates in the head and face, and massage can relieve and soothe away this pressure.

Everyone can benefit from face massage. Men, as much as women, need to have their faces relaxed. Massage can soothe away headaches and eyestrain and give a marvellous feeling of relaxation. This relief of tension not only makes you feel better, but also look better. After a pressure-free holiday you can look ten years younger and the same can happen after a face massage.

The massage stimulates glandular activity and improves the circulation to the skin which helps to prevent the formation of lines and keeps the skin supple, smooth, soft and healthy.

'God hath given you one face, and you make yourself another.'
Hamlet

How to do it

The movements that you use on the face are very similar to those used on the body but obviously they are performed more gently and instead of using the whole hand, you usually use only the fingertips.

Your hands need to be fairly flexible to do face massage, so practise your back massage first. And then when your hands feel more confident move on to the face. Ideally your hands should imperceptibly glide from one movement to the next, from a stimulating movement into a soothing movement without there being a break in the rhythm and without any jerking. Again the basis of a good face massage is rhythm, it should feel like music flowing over the face.

Before you begin

Check your hands. Are your nails short (no hang nails) and your hands clean? Also check that the face you are going to massage is clean, otherwise you will be massaging dirt into the skin.

Your friend can either lie on the floor, or at the foot of the bed with you kneeling (or sitting) behind his or her head.

Use any soft cream or oil for the massage (see some recipes on page 82). Do not use too much cream, just enough so that your fingers are able to move the skin without dragging it.

Some people are scared of face massage. They have the mistaken idea that it can stretch the skin. I find this ridiculous; the skin is strong and resilient. In fact, the opposite applies, for by improving the circulation, you are toning up the muscles and skin with this increase of blood to the tissues. I only have to look at clients who have always had facial massage to verify the truth of this statement. Massage is definitely beneficial to the face.

The face

1. *Stroking the whole face*

Using both hands apply the cream by stroking. Start at the base of the neck and with a large sweeping movement stroke up on either side of the neck. Then from under the chin stroke out under the jaw to the ears, stroke up the sides of the face, up to the temples. Glide down to the chin and starting there stroke up around the mouth, up the sides of the nose, on up the forehead and then out across to each temple. Glide back to the base of the neck. Repeat these two initial stroking movements several times.

This stroking should be very rhythmic, your hands moulding around the contours of the face, applying a little extra pressure on the temples and forehead. One way to get rhythm into your hands is to imagine that your hands are dancing in time to some lovely classical music.

2. *Circles round the chin*
Using your finger tips do upward rotary movements all under the chin and then around each side of the mouth to the nose. Glide back to the chin and then work out across the jawline to the temples. These circles are performed fairly firmly to stimulate the skin.

3. *Finger rolling on the cheeks*
Using the first three fingers of each hand loosely roll them up the cheek. Both hands work on the same side, following each other up alternately. A very stimulating movement.

4. *Finger stroking on the neck*
This is the same as finger rolling, stroking with alternate hands, but this time you work downwards, with both hands on the same side, stroking down the neck, from the chin to the shoulder. You work downwards to help to stimulate the lymphatic drainage system. When you have finished one side, glide over and do the other side.

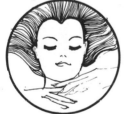

5. *Patting and slapping under the chin*
For this stimulating movement you use the two middle fingers of each hand and 'slap' under the chin and jaw. It is a fast, bouncy movement, stimulating but not heavy. Imagine that you are beating your fingers in time to the music.

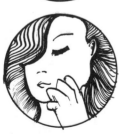

6. *Pinching round the jaw line*
With the thumb and forefinger gently pinch the skin. Pinch under the chin and out under the jaw line, glide back to the chin and pinch out to each temple. This pinching is done fairly fast but be careful, you only want to stimulate, not to leave your poor friend black and blue. This really does help prevent a double chin. I do it when I'm driving and caught in traffic jams.

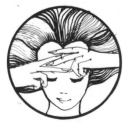

7. *Scissoring across the forehead*
Using your fore and middle fingers in a horizontal position work them across the forehead in a scissor movement. This is a lively fast movement, which helps obliterate those horrible frown lines.

8. *Stroking across the forehead*
From the bridge of the nose draw your fingers out across the forehead to the temples. Give a pressure there and glide back around under the

eyes to the bridge of the nose where you can apply another pressure under the eyebrows there. I finish most of the forehead stroking with pressures at the temples as it is *so* relaxing, and alleviates all the tension that gathers there.

9. *Finger rolling up the forehead*
Stroke firmly up the forehead with your fingers held loosely, rolling and drumming up the forehead. It sounds rather like horses galloping across the forehead and feels marvellous.

10. *Pressures on the forehead*

'An attractive face is the balm of wounded hearts and the key to locked doors.'
Saadi Gulistan, *The Rose Garden*, 1258

Using either your fingers or thumbs (whichever you find the most comfortable), do pressures all over the forehead. Press, release, glide, press, release, glide. It is particularly relaxing to have pressure in the line going up from the nose, especially in the middle on the 'third eye'. The Buddhists believe the 'third eye' to be the seat of the soul. Whether we share their belief or not, it is a very sensitive point and any massage there feels absolutely wonderful.

I use my thumbs to press on the third eye while my fingers also give a light pressure to the temples – it feels incredibly relaxing. Continue these pressures right up to the hairline until you reach the middle of the head.

11. *Stroking round the eyes*
First stroke around both eyes simultaneously and then alternately. You apply the pressure as you massage up and around the eyebrow to the temple, and then glide in towards the nose. I sometimes let one hand follow the other so that it feels like a figure of eight going around the eyes. This is very rhythmic and extremely relaxing. In all these eye movements, be careful not to drag or pull the delicate skin under the eye; you must always glide your finger gently over it, in towards the nose.

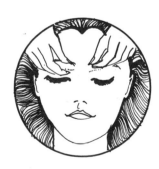

12. *Pinching the eyebrows*
Not surprisingly, there is often a lot of tension around the eyes and this pinching movement is a very effective way of relieving it. Starting at the bridge of the nose, firmly pinch the eyebrow between your thumb and forefinger. Pinch all along the eyebrow and then glide around the eye to start again.

13. *Massaging the eyelid*
Before doing this movement, check that your friend is not wearing contact lenses. (They should have been taken out before you began the face massage.)

Using your ring finger do small gentle rotaries all over the closed eyelid. Finish by giving a long gentle pressure over both eyes simultaneously, pressing down on the eyes with your two middle fingers. Hold the pressure for a second, and then very slowly lift your fingers off to circle the eye. Repeat the whole movement.

14. *The feather touch*

Stroke the forehead with the softest touch possible, hardly touching the skin. This faint, feathery touch is very soothing and relaxing.

Headaches and migraines can be helped by this light, practically imperceptible stroking. Glide your hands gently from the forehead down to the shoulders. When you reach the shoulders shake your hands, as though shaking off water, and start again. Work all over the head and forehead. You can also do this feather touch down the back or even the whole length of the body. It is amazing that this movement, although barely touching the skin, is an effective and almost miraculous cure. It seems too simple to be true, but it really does work, so do try it.

15. *The final touch*

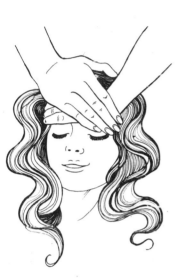

To finish put the palm of one hand on the centre of the forehead and your other hand on top of it. Press down with a firm but even pressure, hold that pressure for a few seconds and then slowly release it. Press, hold, release, press, hold, release. Repeat several times and then gently draw your hands away – and you have finished. Your friend should now be feeling amazingly relaxed and will quite possibly have fallen asleep.

The head

A head massage is the perfect continuation of a face massage, but as there are no large muscles to manipulate on the head it often gets forgotten. Once you have had a head massage you will become addicted. It is *so* relaxing. Head massage is easy to give to friends because they do not have to remove any clothes and can be anywhere. I have often given tired friends head massages at informal parties.

1. *Rotary pressures all over the head*

Using the cushions of your fingers do rotary pressures starting at the hairline, work back to cover the whole head. Actually move the scalp about. If someone is very tense this is practically impossible, but as they relax so does their scalp, and an added bonus is that this scalp massage will stimulate hair growth.

2. *Pressures round the ears*

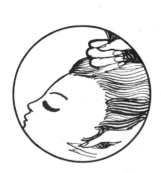

With your thumbs do rotary pressures all around the ears. There are lots of acupuncture points here and it is incredibly relaxing.

Although it sounds crazy, some people even like having the insides of their ears massaged. Try stroking and doing rotaries all around and inside the ear and see if your friend enjoys it.

3. *Pulling the hair!*

Stroke through the hair and firmly clasp a bunch of hair at the roots and give it a steady, gentle pull. Release and move on, pulling the hair all over the head. Although this sounds like something bullies did at school, it has nothing of the bully about it. It just feels as though all the tension is literally being pulled and drawn out. You must try it.

4. *Knuckling the shoulders*
Using your knuckles make small circular movements behind the shoulders, on the fleshy area at the base of the neck. Relax your wrists and make large circles with your knuckles. You can also do this with your fingers. Try both and see which you find the easiest to do.

5. *Alternate stroking up the neck*
Stroke up across the shoulder, and up the neck. Using alternate hands, pull up and stretch the neck, gently pushing the head from side to side. Keep the hands curved and relaxed. Exert a steady pressure with this rhythmic, lazy movement.

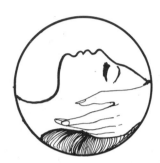

6. *Head rotating*
The head is very heavy, weighing at least six pounds, and it is a lovely feeling to have it supported in someone else's hands, if only for a few minutes.

Support the head with both hands at the base of the skull. Slowly lift the head – not too far, a gentle lifting is enough. Then gently rotate the head, turn it slowly to the right and then over to the left, and then gently lower the head to its original position. Repeat the whole movement twice.

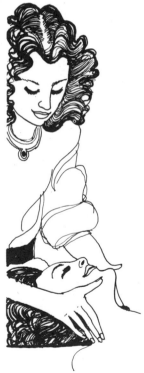

7. *Stretching the neck*
Clasp both your hands behind the head at the base of the skull and with a steady, even pressure, pull the head back towards you. No jerking, just a steady, even pull, then gently release the pressure and replace the head in its original position.

8. *Clasping the head*
Cup your hands on either side of the head, and with your fingers gently covering the ears, firmly press the palms of your hands together. Press, hold, release, press, hold, release. Repeat the pressures several times, gradually moving up to the crown of the head.

9. *The feather touch*
As with the face massage, glide your hand from the forehead and sides of the head through the hair. Repeat gradually getting lighter and lighter.

As you have probably guessed I love head and face massage. It is so relaxing – soothing away worries, headaches and tension, and makes you feel thoroughly pampered – bliss. Aren't cats lucky to have their heads stroked so often?

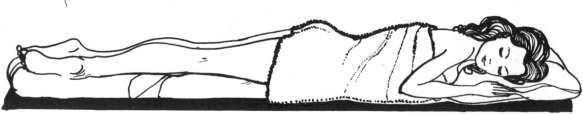

The Three-Week Health Kick

The *Seven-day campaign* should have made you feel fantastic (that is if you stuck to it). You should be full of energy and bursting with health – all ready to continue the good work by following the *Health kick*.

You should still be watching your food intake. Stick to a plain healthy diet. Each day you must keep up doing your daily exercises, your face routine and your body scrubbing. Once each week you should try and have a body or face massage, wash and condition your hair and give yourself a manicure, or pedicure. It is up to you *when* you fit everything in – just as long as you do it all.

The health kick is divided up into weeks one, two and three, and each week has a general theme which is only a rough guide as to how you should be organizing your time. All the facets of your own personalized health and beauty programme have been outlined in *Two-day blitz* and *Seven-day campaign* and the other more detailed chapters. You can make up a three-week programme from merely following the *Seven-day campaign* three times; you could inject a *Two-day blitz* every now and again. But by now you will have acquired the knowledge of the basic principles involved, and can work out your own plan of campaign.

Above all – whichever programme you choose, whether you still have weight to lose or not – the vital points are: Diet, Exercise, General Body and Beauty Care.

Week one

Every day
  (i)   Your daily exercises
 (ii)   Your face; cleansing, toning and creaming
(iii)   Your body; washing, scrubbing and oiling.

Once a week
  (i)   Your face and body massage
 (ii)   Your hair conditioning and washing
(iii)   Your manicure and pedicure.

Start the week by weighing and measuring yourself – and do the mirror test to show what a difference this healthy life makes and also to see how wonderful you are looking!

Week One has the general theme of the health of your body which involves many things. Firstly must come *Diet*. You should still be watching your diet and sticking to a simple low calorie routine. For this first week I have made lists of all the foods you are allowed to eat, about 1,000 calories per day. Nutritionally, this will provide you with everything that your body needs.

You can eat the food how and when you like, and you will find that it will give you a great choice of meals. I have not allowed for drinks, so if you are going out give yourself an allowance of 200 calories.

Every day
Remember to drink at least 4–8 glasses of water. Drink as much herb tea as you wish but try to cut down on coffee and ordinary tea. Use our Low Calorie Salad dressing on all the salads. If you want to substitute one food for another, check its calorie value either from the lists in the *Seven-day campaign*, or buy a little pocket calorie counting book and refer to that. I use the *Complete Calorie Counter* which was brought out by *Slimming Magazine* and is very comprehensive.

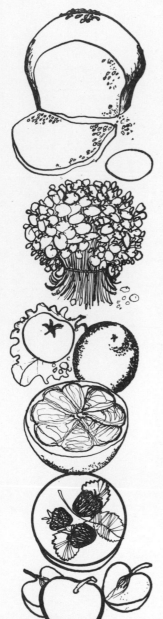

Week One Diet

Day 1
½ pt/300 ml skimmed low fat milk
½ oz/15 g butter or margarine
1 slice wholemeal bread
Our Health Cereal
1 egg
4 oz/100 g lean grilling steak
1 bunch watercress
½ cucumber
½ lettuce
1 tomato
8 oz/200 g spinach
1 orange
½ grapefruit
1 apple or 4 oz/100 g strawberries

Day 2
1 pt/300 ml low fat milk
½ oz/15 g butter or margarine
1 slice wholemeal bread
1 egg
6 oz/175 g chicken joint
6 oz/175 g white fish
1 small carton low fat yoghurt
4 oz/100 g green beans
4 oz/100 g cabbage
Celery
2 carrots
2 tomatoes
1 orange
1 apple or pear
½ oz/15 g raisins

Day 3
½ pt/300 ml low fat milk
½ oz/15 g butter or margarine
1 slice wholemeal bread
Our Health Cereal
2 oz/50 g hard cheese
    (or 4 oz/100 g chicken livers)
8 oz/200 g mackerel (baked)
    or sardines
4 oz/100 g consommé
2 tomatoes
½ bunch watercress
4 oz/100 g cabbage
½ lettuce
1 cucumber
1 onion
1 orange

Day 4
½ pt/300 ml low fat milk
½ oz/15 g butter or margarine
1 slice wholemeal bread
1 egg
4 oz/100 g cottage cheese
6–7 oz/175–200 g chicken
    drumsticks
1 aubergine (approx. 6 oz/175 g)
4 oz/100 g courgettes
1 green pepper
1 onion
1 tomato
1 small baked potato
3 oz/75 g bean sprouts
2 oranges
4 oz/100 g slice melon

Day 5
½ pt/300 ml low fat milk
½ oz/15 g butter or margarine
1 slice wholemeal bread
Our Health Cereal
1 lean lamb chop (or ¼ lb/100 g liver)
6 oz/175 g white fish
4 oz/100 g mushrooms
½ bunch watercress
¼ cauliflower
1 apple or grapefruit
1 orange

Day 6
½ pt/300 ml low fat milk
½ oz/15 g butter or margarine
1 slice wholemeal bread
1 egg
4 oz/100 g drained tuna fish
6 oz/175 g chicken
4 oz/100 g consommé
½ lettuce
1 tomato
1 green pepper
1 onion
4 oz/100 g green beans
1 orange
1 grapefruit

Day 7
½ pt/300 ml low fat milk
½ oz/15 g butter or margarine
1 slice wholemeal bread
Our Health Cereal
1 egg
2 slices lean ham
4 oz/100 g grilling steak

8 oz/225 g spinach
4 oz/100 g mushrooms
2 tomatoes
¼ cauliflower
1 apple or peach
½ grapefruit

Isometrics (or exercises you can do anywhere)

Paramount to the health of our bodies is exercise, and for your 'daily dozen' do refer again (if you need!) to the *Exercises* chapter (pages 145–58). You really ought to be aware of your body all the time. What do you do for the main bulk of the day? Sit in an office, do the house-work, cook or rush around after a family? Whatever it is, then is when you could (and should) be doing some exercises during that time. Train yourself to utilize your body properly all the time; think of your muscles and remember to use them – pull them in, push them up, tense and relax them, work the muscles against each other.

When you are sitting, either at home or work, remember to sit up straight. Never slump into a chair with a curved back and relaxed tummy. Instead, actually use the muscles in your stomach and back and sit straight. Stretch when making the beds, or reaching for the telephone. Remember to bend your knees when picking anything up. Make sure that you are working in conditions that you find comfortable. Is your chair the correct height for you? Can you reach the ironing board easily? Be constantly aware of, and use, your body.

I know someone who conducts million dollar deals on the floor. Her office has telephones and piles of papers all over the floor. She used to suffer from back ache and found that if she worked on the floor she was comfortable. Although she does absolutely no energetic exercise (she rarely even walks) her muscles are in extremely good shape, because

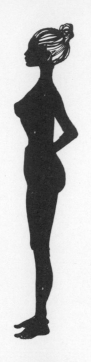

she is using them all the time; she sits, she kneels on all fours, she stretches and gets up and down. All this gentle, but continual, exercise is enough for her body and she even went from 11 stone to 9 stone and retained a firm, shapely figure.

How to have a flat stomach
There are simply hundreds of exercises for flattening the stomach, but the very best is this one, which can be done anywhere and at any time. It is almost too simple to write down. We all know this exercise but we forget about it, and perhaps don't realize how effective it is. I was reminded of it by a client who said that after her fifth child she was so disgusted with her 'wobbly stomach', she became fanatical about remembering to use her tummy muscles. She pulled them in at every opportunity, and had soon retrained them (she has a marvellous flat and firm stomach).

It couldn't be easier, just pull in your stomach, hold it in for the count of 20 (remember to keep on breathing) and then slowly relax the muscles. You can vary the length you hold them in, just hold it for as long as you feel comfortable.

This really is one of the exercises you can do *anywhere* and at *anytime*. There is really no excuse not to do it. Do it now as you are reading – pull those muscles right in, hold them in, and then slowly release. Repeat frequently.

The side effect of this exercise is that you will not only have a flat stomach, it will also improve your posture.

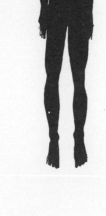

Aching back and round shoulders
If you suffer from either of these then try and do this simple exercise. Next time you are slumped over a book or slouched over the cooking, relax for an instant and hunch your shoulders up towards your ears, hold, then relax, then pull them backwards, again hold and relax. Do this whenever you remember and you will be amazed to find that it really does help. The efficacy of this exercise was proved to me by a friend who had extremely round shoulders and had a permanent back ache. She started doing it whilst reading in the library and noticed an almost miraculous improvement.

Most back troubles – and they're as common as the common cold – are caused by weakness in the muscles and ligaments. If you strengthen these back muscles – and your stomach muscles too curiously enough – you should never suffer a bad back again. Lack of control of the stomach and back muscles can cause an imbalance in the body which results in some muscles being over-used and others being under-used and this leads to fatigue, tension and pain. It's all a case of learning to use your body correctly.

If you feel tension accumulating, try some relaxing exercises (see page 155) or rest on your slant board (see page 68), do gentle exercises for 5–10 minutes per day (see particularly exercises 3, 12 and 13 on pages 148 and 150–51).

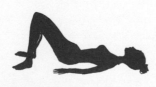

Another marvellous way to relieve an aching back is again incredibly simple. Lie on your back, flat on the floor with your knees up and your feet on the floor. Put a couple of books under your head so that it is in line with your body. Just lie there and gradually the tension will leave your muscles and your back will straighten out. Lie like this for at least 10 minutes, and do this exercise twice a day. I know it sounds almost *too* easy but it really does help.

Slim ankles

A client recently told me that when she was young she complained to her beautician that she had greasy skin and fat ankles. She was told that she was lucky as 'Women with greasy skin and fat ankles end up with no lines and slim ankles, whereas those with dry skin and thin ankles will have lined faces and matchstick ankles'! If you don't look after your skin, that is certainly true, but the theory about the ankles seems to be wishful thinking.

However, this same woman told me that she eventually found a way to slim her ankles. She moved to a flat on the fourth floor of an old building without a lift. After a few weeks of going up and down 196 steps at least four times a day she found that a miracle had taken place – her ankles were slim. So if you want slim ankles forget the lift, and walk up and down the stairs!

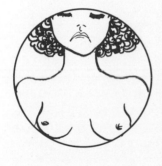

A firm bust

It's possible to strengthen the supporting muscles of the bust whilst doing something else. Contract the side muscles of your neck (it is easy if you pull the sides of your mouth down) and you will see and feel your bust moving. This helps firm up the bust. I try just to exercise these muscles without pulling my mouth down (I'm not crazy about the idea of having my face in that position – the wind might change and I might stay like that!).

The purpose of all these examples is to make you aware of your muscles. Decide which *you* need, and incorporate these easy movements into your life. I spend a lot of my time driving and so do them whilst sitting in the car. I pull in my tummy, tense up my buttocks, and exercise my bust muscles whilst waiting in traffic jams, and so, if you see someone grimacing and bouncing up and down in a car, it will probably be me!

Cellulite

This word, which strikes horror into the hearts of those of us who are even a tiny bit overweight or over 30, was coined by the French and refers to the puckered, unhealthy looking fat which sometimes accumulates on women's thighs and men's stomachs. Thin people, as well as fat, can suffer from this complaint and I have even noticed children with it. It is usually caused by bad circulation and fluid retention. The fatty tissue contains too much moisture, giving an orange-peel appearance to the skin. Confusion can sometimes arise because there is an English word 'cellulitis' which refers to a medical condition, an acute inflammation of the skin. But when I mention cellulite I am referring to the French word.

The way to tackle the problem is to improve your diet, and to increase the circulation to the area by massage and exercise. Massage with a string glove or loofah, and then use the kneading movements described on page 90. Massage really firmly to tone up the skin and muscles. Exercise as much as possible as this will both improve the muscle tone and circulation. Running a cold shower over the area also helps – again it stimulates the circulation.

Watch your diet, to try and prevent water retention, cut out sugar and eat as little starch as possible. Eat lots of green vegetables instead.

If you exercise and massage yourself daily you really will find that the unsightly 'bobbly' fat will diminish – and disappear. It is worth that extra bit of effort to achieve this result.

I read recently that kelp helps to diminish water retention, fat and cellulite (it is often one of the ingredients in 'anti-cellulite' creams). I have not been able to test its efficacy yet, but it is certainly worth a try. You could also make the salt body scrub on page 69.

Patchouli oil is also thought to help in the fight against water retention. Try massaging yourself with this oil. Shake the oils together in a small bottle and use at least once, preferably twice, daily. Massage it well into the problem area.

4 tablespoons sunflower oil (about 2 fl. ozs.)
1 tablespoon wheatgerm oil
½ teaspoon patchouli oil

Passive muscle exercisers

Another method of toning up muscles is 'Slendertone'. Although I am a tremendous advocate of active exercise, I think that this passive muscle exercising method is extremely useful. It is especially good for spot reducing, or for getting back into shape after pregnancy.

These machines work on the faradic principle, sending an alternating current through to the muscle so that it contracts and relaxes. Pads are placed on the muscles, the machine is switched on, and the muscles are made to contract and relax at the equivalent of about 1,000 exercises each half hour, which is obviously far more concentrated exercise than you could do yourself in that time – and with no effort! You would have to exercise for hours to achieve the same results. For those times when you have neglected your exercises – and your body shows this slackness – these machines are extremely useful. Just before the summer holidays when bikinis are tried on again, my beauty practise becomes extremely busy giving these treatments. They definitely do tone up the muscles and firm the body. And, after the treatments hopefully the clients will keep their now firm, lithe bodies in shape for the rest of the summer (and year) by doing their exercises.

I also find that the use of these machines is particularly successful on the muscles of the abdomen that are stretched during pregnancy. If a woman exercises immediately after childbirth, her stomach muscles will go back into shape quickly and effectively, but so often at that time, women are extremely busy and too tired to exercise enough, and so then this passive muscle exerciser is a most effective treatment.

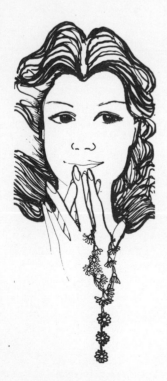

Your bust

When you're looking after your body and its health – as you are this week – you mustn't forget about your bust.

Weight loss can cause a reduction in the size of the bust and so you need to pay particular attention to keeping it firm. Exercise is extremely important to strengthen the pectoral muscles (see page 150). Massage is also useful – do stimulating movements all over the upper part of the bust. Gently pat and tap between the breasts and up to the base of the neck and beginning of the shoulders. Lightly massage around the base of your breast towards the nipple.

An Oriental client told me that the best treatment for the bust was to splash it with cold water. She keeps a round bowl about the size of her bust in the bathroom which she fills with cold water and then cups her bust with this. If her bust is anything to go by this simple treatment is definitely worth copying. A few years ago the French brought out a 'bust firmer' which was based on this simple theory.

A marvellous recipe for a bust tonic was given to me by a Belgian client who swears by it. Mix 2 oz/50 g of good lard with about $\frac{1}{4}$ to $\frac{1}{2}$ dl of white wine vinegar. Add the vinegar to the lard slowly as though you were making mayonnaise. Massage this 'bust tonic' into the bust every day.

Hands and legs

1 egg yolk
2 teaspoons ground almonds
1 teaspoon honey
1 teaspoon almond oil

After your bust, you might spare a thought for your hands and your legs. If your hands are chapped, parched or just in thoroughly bad condition, then they need a hand mask. Mix these ingredients together into a paste and apply, then put on some cotton or kid gloves. The gloves keep the mask in place and the heat will help the hands absorb the mask. I frequently use this hand mask after too much gardening (without gloves on!). I also apply it to my feet which, due to the fact that I am always barefoot, can always do with extra pampering. It leaves the hands (and feet) beautifully soft, white and smooth.

Hand masks and 'sleeping gloves' used to be worn in bed by women in Tudor times, thus conditioning their hands while they slept. In *Aids to Health and Beauty*, 1898, I found this recipe: 'An excellent preparation for your sleeping gloves. Hands that are inclined to chap should be rubbed frequently with a paste of a spoonful of honey and two of fine oatmeal. Beat these up with the yolks of two eggs and add sufficient unsalted. lard to make a paste; thoroughly mix all together. This preparation will be excellent for smearing your sleeping gloves with.'

NO. 6 HAND AND BODY LOTION

1 tablespoon stearic acid
$\frac{1}{2}$ teaspoon emulsifying wax
2 tablespoons sunflower oil
5 tablespoons boiled water or rose water
1 teaspoon glycerine
2 drops orange-flower oil

This is another invaluable cream for softening the skin on both hands and body – an improved version of the old-fashioned glycerine and rose water lotion our grandmothers used to make.

Melt the waxes and oils in a bowl in a water bath and in a separate bowl heat the water and glycerine to the same temperature. When the waxes are melted remove them from the heat and slowly add the water and glycerine stirring continuously until the cream becomes cool. I use my electric beater on the low speed and soon have about half a cup of fine pearly cream. It is the stearic acid which makes the cream look pearly and which also gives a lovely, satin sheen to the skin.

I called the cream No. 6 because when I experiment I number all my creams and then ask friends to sample them and see which they

½ pt/300 ml sunflower oil
3 tablespoons crushed
   rosemary
2 tablespoons crushed
   lavender
1 tablespoon vodka

prefer – and this, number six of that day's experimenting, was chosen.

Leg oil. If you ever suffer from aching legs, try this beautifully smelling oil. Several clients have found that if they massage their legs with this oil every day, it relieves the aching. Mix everything together and use.

Week two

Don't forget

Every day
  (i)   Your daily exercises
  (ii) Your face cleaning, toning and creaming
 (iii) Your body washing, scrubbing and oiling

Once a week
  (i)   Your face and body massage
  (ii) Your hair conditioning and washing
 (iii) Your manicure and pedicure

Once again, exactly how you plan this middle week of your *Three-week health kick* is up to you. You must remember all the details listed above and you must stay on a restricted diet (I outline another approach this week which may appeal to you more). This week's general theme is care of the body and don't forget to turn to the chapters on skin and hair etc. to fill in any gaps.

The sociable diet

At about this time in any regime, boredom can set in; hopefully you have been dieting successfully on our low calorie diet, and are probably ready for a change. With our 'sociable diet' – carbohydrate counting – you can re-enter your busy social life with complete confidence, and no one need know you are on a diet. So for the rest of the *Health kick* I suggest you switch to the 'Low Carbohydrate Diet'. This is the diet that you can easily maintain for the rest of your life.

    You will find that a low carbohydrate diet will also cut down your calorie intake. In fact, the diets I have outlined in my 'campaigns' have not only been cutting down on calories – they have also been low in carbohydrates. We have been trying to change our eating habits, so that we always eat a really healthy, nutritious diet.

    On a low carbohydrate diet you are allowed to eat as much fat as you like. Some people think that this will make them put on weight, but by cutting out all the carbohydrates and the hidden fat they contain (in biscuits, cakes etc.) you will find that you probably also decrease the amount of fat you eat. Without bread you'll eat less butter and jam, without puddings you'll eat less cream. Eating some fat, however, stops you feeling hungry as it goes through the stomach slower than other food and makes you feel full for longer. Without fat, you can also feel irritated, and the skin can suffer.

    The average intake of carbohydrate is about 400 grams a day and

'The best cosmetic is happiness and good health.'
Queen Christina of
Sweden, born 1626

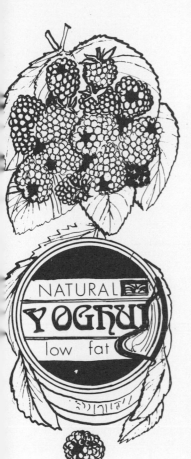

so if this is reduced to 60 or 80 grams you are bound to lose weight. In most charts of food values the food is calculated in grams per ounce (25 g). But I think it is easier if I give the carbohydrate value of an average portion. Most of us would eat a whole apple (not an ounce) which would weigh roughly 4 oz/100 g, so in the lists that follow I will give the value of an average portion.

The lists of food are there for you to refer to initially, but very quickly you will have learnt what you can eat to your heart's content, and what you should avoid.

FOODS TO EAT WHENEVER YOU WISH
There are plenty of foods which contain absolutely no carbohydrate: meat, fish, poultry, sardines, cheese, margarine, butter and oil. You can also fill yourself up on green vegetables, cauliflower, salad and eggs because they only contain a trace amount.

FOODS TO EAT IN MODERATION
Fruit, tomatoes, yoghurt, cottage cheese, bread, peas, pulses, corn and nuts. Although milk is fairly high in carbohydrate it should not be eliminated. You should drink about ½ pint/300 ml a day to ensure that you have a nutritionally balanced diet.

FOODS TO AVOID
Pasta, flour, root vegetables, cereals, biscuits, cakes, dried mixes and fruit juices, bananas and dried fruit, sausages.

ALCOHOL
On a sociable diet you are probably going to want to have the occasional drink. Although alcohol does not actually contain carbohydrate it does contain sorbitol (which gives the drink its sweetness), and for the purpose of our diet, we must count this as being the equivalent of carbohydrates. One ounce/15 g of alcohol gives you about 20 grams of carbohydrates.

Planning your meals when you are carbohydrate counting is really easy – there is just so much choice. Here is an easy guide line.

Breakfast		*Carbohydrates*
½ grapefruit	5 ⎫	
1 egg and 1 rasher bacon	⎬	20
Slice wholemeal bread	15 ⎭	
Our Health Cereal (see page 63)		20

Main meal
Consommé, asparagus, meat, fish, poultry, vegetables (especially green), cheese and salad (trace)

Light meal
Meat, fish, poultry or eggs
Vegetables or salad
Piece of fruit   10–20

Unfortunately fruit contains a fairly large quantity of carbohydrate – due to its sugar content – and so eat fruit in moderation. As an example, here is the carbohydrate value of average portions of fruit (100 g) and of juices.

Apple	10	Strawberries	6
Apricots (dried, about 6 halves)	10	1 oz/25 g raisins	
Avocado pear ($\frac{1}{2}$)	5	and sultanas	20
Banana	19	Canned fruit juices	15
Orange	10	Apple juice	11
Peach	10	Orange juice	10

What is really wonderful about this diet is that one can be so sociable. No more avoiding dinner parties or restaurants, no one need even guess you are on a diet – so eat (carbohydrateless-ly) and become slim.

A friend of mine who has just lost three-quarters of a stone in a fortnight on this carbohydrate counting diet tells me how important and helpful a tool your weighing machine is. He weighed himself at the same time each day; when there was a weight loss this encouraged him to keep to the diet, and when there wasn't he adjusted his eating that day and cut down.

If you become really interested in this form of slimming, I suggest that you read Professor Yudkin's marvellous book *This Slimming Business* (Penguin, 1962). Or buy a handy little pocket book with the carbohydrate values of all food. There are several on the market. I used the *Complete Carbohydrate Counter* (Pan, 1978).

Hair
I have discussed hair care in a number of other places (see pages 27 and 75), but these are a few other aspects which you may be interested in trying, and which at least, I hope, will amuse you!

LANOLIN SHAMPOO

½ teaspoon lanolin
1 teaspoon sunflower oil
2 tablespoons water
2 tablespoons clear
shampoo

It's time to wash your hair again, why not try using this shampoo which both conditions and adds body, and so is marvellous for dry, or fine, flyaway hair. Simply melt the lanolin, add the oil to that, and then beat in the water and shampoo.

DRY SHAMPOO
Occasionally you just don't have the time to wash your hair, and so dry shampoos are extremely useful. The best that I have tried is Orris root powder (available from any good health shop or herbalist).

Part your hair and apply the powder sparingly. Brush it through your hair and continue brushing until you've removed all traces of it. The mistake most people make when using a dry shampoo is to apply too much which means that it is almost impossible to remove and the hair ends up looking chalky instead of dirty – so apply a little at a time.

Orris root has a beautiful delicate smell and so it will not only leave your hair looking clean, it also leaves it smelling clean.

'A great lady wrote "Satan smells of sulphur, and I smell of orris root"; she could not have chosen a more exquisite odour' – Lady Colin Campbell, *The Lady's Dressing Room*, London 1892.

Rinses

The hair washing routine can be improved by one of these hair rinses. In the *Two-day blitz* we used diluted vinegar and lemon juice, but this week we shall use herbs as well.

Rosemary is renowned for its use as a hair conditioner, and is said to stimulate hair growth and prevent premature baldness. Simmer a handful of rosemary in a cup of red vinegar. Strain and bottle the mixture and when you use it, dilute about $\frac{1}{4}$ cup with a cup of water. This diluted rosemary-vinegar makes a marvellous final hair rinse which leaves the hair with a lovely sheen.

Rosemary enjoys the reputation of 'strengthening the brain' which could be the reason that it became the emblem of fidelity for lovers. Chamomile is also well known in connection with hair and continued use of it helps keep fair hair blonde. Simmer two tablespoons of chamomile in a cup of white wine vinegar. Bottle the mixture and dilute it for use as above. It leaves the hair looking beautifully shiny and full of highlights.

The following, more exotic version is from an old Flemish manuscript. Make the hair rinse in the same method as the previous two recipes; simmer all the ingredients together, strain them and bottle the liquid, diluting it as above.

By using a final hair rinse, you remove all traces of soap scum, restore the hair's acidity and leave the hair more manageable and lustrous.

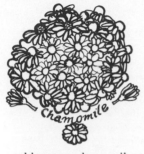

2 tablespoons chamomile
3 tablespoons rose petals
(white)
1 tablespoon marjoram
1 cup wine vinegar

Conditioners

Everyone's hair can benefit from conditioning. If your hair is dry you must try and counteract this dryness. But conditioning can also help greasy hair as some conditioners not only oil the hair, they also cleanse and treat it.

YOGHURT

I learnt about the use of yoghurt as a hair conditioner from a young mountaineer in Afghanistan. He said that it was the very best way of both conditioning the hair, and preventing dandruff. I have frequently used it since then and found that it does make the hair beautifully shiny. Simply massage the yoghurt in, leave it for about 10–20 minutes, rinse it out, and then wash your hair.

MASHED AVOCADO

*'A woman who cannot be ugly
is not beautiful.'*
Karl Kraus

This also makes a terrific hair conditioner (and face mask). Use it by itself or add it to your 'mayonnaise' (see page 22). Again leave it on for about 10–20 minutes, rinse it out and wash your hair in the normal way.

Hair 'restoring'

After all the love and attention you have been lavishing on your hair it should now be looking beautifully shiny, but for some of us that is not enough. We would like to have *more* hair. Here are some ways to encourage it. '*To Quicken the Growth of Hair. Dip the teeth of your comb, every morning in the expressed juice of nettles and comb the hair the wrong way.*' *Toilet of Flora, 1784*

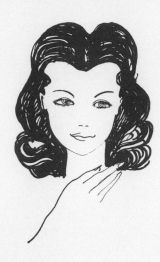

Nettles, as the above shows, have always been used as a hair tonic. Here is a recipe I have found effective. Simmer a handful of chopped, fresh nettles in equal parts of water and white wine vinegar (about ½ cup of each) for about 20 minutes and then strain. It has a slightly unattractive smell and so I add a couple of drops of rosemary oil which is a stimulant and very good for the hair. Massage the tonic into the scalp every day and you should soon notice an improvement.

The only problem with nettles is their sting. As Culpeper said, 'They need no description, they can be found by feeling on the darkest night'. To avoid this problem remember to wear gloves when picking them and when making the hair tonic!

The remedy that I have found most effective for encouraging hair growth – and as a fantastic hair conditioner – is the use of marrowbone. All you need is a large bone. Scoop the marrow out, melt it, and apply the resulting oily fat onto your scalp. Massage it in well and then wrap your head in kitchen foil and keep it on for as long as possible.

The woman who originally told me about this treatment used it every day for a week. She applied it in the evening and kept it on all night. The results were miraculous. Her hair had been in terrible condition and was steadily getting thinner and thinner. With the treatment, she noticed an improvement after only a few days.

Since putting this recipe in my last book, I have heard from many readers of the effectiveness of this treatment. So, although it is a time-consuming and rather messy treatment, I *do* recommend it. It really is the very best hair conditioner I know, leaving the hair feeling silky, and looking thick and lustrous.

Onion juice applied to the scalp is said to encourage growth. It is also a strong antiseptic and can be applied practically anywhere. As Culpeper tells us, 'The juice of onions used with malt vinegar takes away all blemishes, spots and marks in the skin, and dropped in the ears eases the pains and noises of them'.

Lotions which when applied to the hair will cause miraculous hair growth have long been in existence. In the Victorian era especially, they abounded. Here's an extract from the advertisement for Koko Hair Lotion which 'Eradicates Scurf, Promotes Growth, Prevents Hair Falling. Will Positively Stop Hair from Falling Out and Prevent it turning Prematurely Grey. Will certainly increase the Growth of the Hair, and if constantly used will make it Bright, Soft and Wavy. . . . The best plan is to apply Koko freely, and brush the scalp until a warm glow is produced'.

A bottle containing 12½ fluid ounces cost 4/6d (22½p). When it was analysed it was found to contain borax, glycerine, perfume, alcohol, formaldehyde solution and water. And that 12½ ounces cost one penny!

Things haven't changed much! We are still being offered lotions and potions of all descriptions which sound fantastic and exciting and achieve very little.

Perhaps The Empress Dowager of China, Tz'u-li, known as The Dragon Empress, might have taken advantage of some of these potions:

'The years that a woman subtracts from her age are not lost. They are added to other women's.'
Diane de Poitiers

'. . . (she) was scrupulous in her attention to detail. She had the grey streaks in her hair dyed black. It stained her scalp as well in those days, and in later years she was delighted when a dye from Paris was procured which left the skin white.

'Once, when as a young girl, she was having her hair combed by a eunuch his hand shook, and he combed out three black hairs in the comb. "Put Them Back. *PUT THEM BACK!*" shrieked Tz'u-li. She was only placated when it was suggested to her that he should be beaten to death.'

Marina Warner, *The Dragon Empress*,
Weidenfeld & Nicolson, 1972

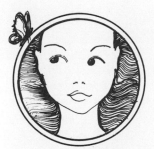

Eyes

'Fair was the day but fairer was the maid,
Who that day's morn into the greenwood strayed.
Sweet was her breathing,
Such rare perfumes the roses are bequeathing.
Bright shone the sunne, but brighter were her eyes,
Such are the lamps that guide the deities.

William Browne, 1590–1643

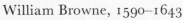

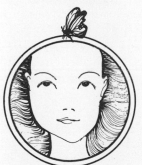

As we continue with our beauty week, we must not forget about our eyes. The prerequisite for shining, bright eyes is health. If you have been following your diet, drinking lots of water, having lots of fresh air, and doing all the exercises I have been advising throughout the weeks, then your eyes should be sparkling with health. Eyes, more than anything else, reflect the way you feel: dull and listless when you're depressed or run-down, and 'starry-eyed' when you're healthy and happy. Lack of sleep, too much smoking, indigestion and excessive alcohol are all instantly reflected by eyes which lack lustre or are red and puffy. Sleep is the most important factor towards beautiful, clear eyes and so make sure that you are getting enough. You automatically rest your eyes during the day by blinking and you can consciously improve on this natural way of relaxing by 'palming'. Close your eyes and cover them with your hands, the right palm slightly cupped over the right eye and the left palm over the left eye. Relax like that for a couple of minutes and when you remove your hands you should feel tremendously refreshed.

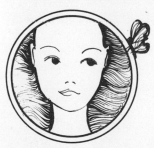

Eye exercises
Exercising your eyes is as important as exercising any other part of the body. Blink, look from side to side, roll your eyes around, look at the four corners of the room and wiggle your forehead. All these simple eye movements will strengthen the eyes, and with luck, postpone the need for glasses.

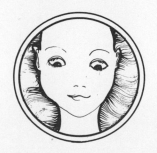

Eye lotions and pads
It is marvellously relaxing to lie down for a few minutes with eye pads on your eyes – the total darkness refreshes one's mind and the wet pads relieve any tiredness from the eyes.

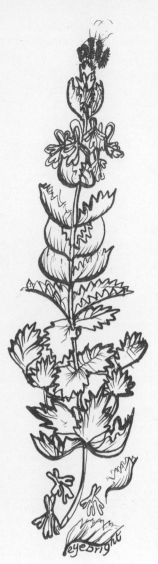

eyebright

Eyebright, as its name suggests, makes the most wonderful eye lotion and Culpeper has this to say about it: 'If the herb was but half as much used as it is neglected, it would half spoil the spectacle makers' trade and a man would think that reason should teach people to prefer the preservation of their natural sight before artificial spectacles, which they may be instructed how to do, take the virtues of *Eyebright* as followeth: The juice or distilled water of Eyebright taken inwardly with white wine, or broth, or dropped into the eyes for several days together helpeth all infirmities of the eye that causes dimness of sight.' He went on to say that it also strengthened the brain and memory. All of these reasons point out the usefulness of this herb. Here's my recipe for the eye lotion.

Pour a pint of boiling water over two tablespoons of eyebright (dried). Cover the container and allow the infusion to stand for two hours. Strain it twice through filter paper and then add one tablespoon of witch hazel. Keep it in a capped bottle and use as often as you wish. Cotton wool pads soaked in this eye lotion make marvellous eye pads to use when you relax with your face mask during a facial.

Cold tea also makes an excellent eye lotion. Try using dampened tea bags on your eyes when you relax.

Cucumber slices are well-known used as eye pads – they always feel so cool and refreshing.

Potato slices can also be used, and crazy as it sounds, make very good eye pads – they seem to relieve puffy eyes and diminish bags under the eyes.

Rotten apples are used in some parts of England as a poultice in a remedy for sore eyes.

The Scandinavian Gods kept themselves ever young by eating apples of Idun, Goddess of Youth and Spring. In Welsh legends kings and heroes go to live happily after death to a paradise of apple trees called Avalon. The apple probably owes its connection with immortality to its colour. Wild apples (crab apples) and many other apples turn red and yellow as they ripen, and these are the colours of the sun, which rises new and living again with each new morning. Perhaps this is the origin of the ancient saying 'An apple a day keeps the doctor away'.

Cold water makes a very effective eye tonic. Whenever you wash your face, cup your hands, fill them with cold water and bathe your eyes with it. Gently splash the water onto your eyes. Repeat this about ten times.

This is a marvellous way to wake yourself up, or to refresh tired eyes. It leaves your eyes toned up, glowing and clear.

Eyebrows

Eyebrows – 'those Cupid groves of delight' as Mrs Beeton so eloquently referred to them in 1694 – should frame and enhance your eyes. Whether eyebrows are thick or thin is largely dictated by fashion and nationality. For instance in some parts of the world it is considered a sign of beauty if your eyebrows meet in the middle. But the general consensus is that eyebrows should start on a line from the tear duct and end at an angle up from the outer corner of the eye. It is easy to

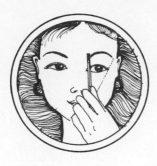

see this arch, if you take a pencil and hold it next to the nose pointing up the forehead. The eyebrow should start on that line, then turn the pencil so that one end is next to the nose and the other by the outer corner of the eye and up to where the eyebrow should end.

To pluck your eyebrows first brush them into the shape you desire (a child's small toothbrush is ideal for this). And then, following your natural line pluck from underneath. Be careful, take one hair out at a time and occasionally brush them into shape again. Brush, pluck, brush, pluck. Once you have taken one too many out you can't do anything about the hole and so your eyebrows will either look moth eaten or become thinner and thinner. So pluck with care!

When you've finished plucking wipe your eyebrows with witch hazel or a skin tonic – don't forget to clean your tweezers and occasionally sterilize them with some alcohol.

> *'When the eye is pure it sees purity.'*
> Hakim Sani: *The Walled Garden of Truth*

Eyelashes

Don't forget to put cream on your eyelashes. Mascara tends to be drying and so they need an occasional 'oiling'.

I have frequently been told that vaseline applied to the eyelashes makes them grow. When I tried it I never noticed any difference, but it's always worth a try.

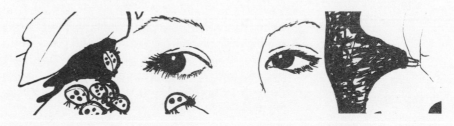

Baths

The beautifying and relaxing of your body is the theme for this week, and nothing works such wonders as a candlelit bath. I discovered the bliss of bathing by candlelight purely by accident. London was having electricity power cuts and there was no choice. How glad I am.

Fill the bath with warm water and your favourite bath oil, and light the room with a candle (maybe even a scented one). Put on your favourite music so that it too can waft over you. Shut the door of the bathroom and *relax*. Day dream and lose yourself to the world. (You can practically imagine all those exciting events in the adverts coming true – maybe somebody actually will arrive with a box of chocolates, a bottle of vodka, or a white horse.)

Bath oils

These bath oils are essentially aromatic. The oil makes a film on top of the water so that when you are in the bath you can lie back and enjoy its delicate fragrance. The oil clings to the body when you get out and so let as much as possible remain on the skin by patting yourself dry.

Mix all the ingredients together in a bottle (there's enough for several baths).

1. FLORAL BATH OIL	2. REFRESHER BATH OIL	3. ORIENTAL BATH OIL
1 oz/25 g almond or sunflower oil	1 oz/25 g almond or sunflower oil	1 oz/25 g almond or sunflower oil
12 drops rose oil	3 drops bergamot oil	12 drops sandalwood oil
3 drops honey-suckle oil	6 drops rosemary oil	4 drops musk oil
9 drops jasmin oil	12 drops lavender oil	8 drops amber oil
		10 drops jasmin oil

I have suggested the number of drops to an ounce of oil but these are only suggestions. Some oils are stronger than others and you might like a very aromatic bath whereas someone else would like a delicately fragrant bath. Adjust the recipes to suit yourself, and make up your own personal favourite.

Bath salts

Bath salts soften, scent and colour the water and can make your bath more exciting and enjoyable. They are extremely easy to make. All you need is approximately 1 lb/450 g sodium sesqui carbonate, food colouring and your favourite perfume (pine or eucalyptus are mine).

Put the sodium sesqui carbonate into a large bowl, add the colouring drop by drop, and mix it in by hand until you have an even colour. Wear rubber gloves as this can cause irritation. Then mix in the perfume, and you have made enough bath salts to last you for months (packets of your own bath salts make marvellous presents).

The sodium sesqui carbonate can be ordered from your local chemist. You will usually have to buy a fairly large quantity – but it is relatively cheap. You will find that these bath salts are as good as any you could buy and they work out infinitely cheaper.

Bubble baths

1 egg
1 tablespoon clear gelatine
1 cup cheap clear shampoo
½ teaspoon essential oil

Soak away any tiredness or stiffness in a lovely, long, luxurious bubble bath. For this first recipe, beat the egg and slowly add in the liquid shampoo then sprinkle on the gelatine and continue beating. To make sure it sets put this mixture over a water bath for about 10 minutes and it will gel. Add in the essential oil, lemon verbena or lavender, which will make it smell beautifully refreshing. Put about a tablespoon of the gel into the bath when the water is running, and there you are with a beautiful bubble bath.

2½ cups Teepol
2 tablespoons gum arabic or gum tragacanth
¼ cup glycerine
3 tablespoons Saponin
3 teaspoons pine oil

This next version gives a bubble bath which is indistinguishable from the commercial ones; but the problem is that the ingredients are a little difficult to obtain. Teepol is the base for washing-up liquid. Saponin is a foam stabilizer which is quite dangerous, and so great care should be taken when using it. It is also a little difficult to obtain. I suggest that you mix the ingredients together outside and protect your hands with rubber gloves.

Mix the Teepol, glycerine and gum arabic together in a large bowl and then add in the saponin, stirring one tablespoon in at a time so that the powder doesn't become lumpy – or, you can put all the ingredients into a large wide necked jar and shake them together.

Add in the pine oil (or any scent you particularly like) and I also add in a little colouring – green if you are using pine or cochineal if you're using rose – it's fun experimenting with different food colouring.

Bubble baths are real morale boosters. It is such a luxurious feeling sitting in all these bubbles – just like being a Hollywood film-star of the 20's.

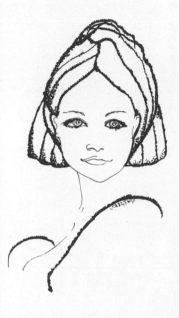

Turkish bath

You could also try at some time in the week having a Turkish bath or sauna. There is nothing quite as pampering – all that heat enveloping you and simply forcing you to relax. The principle of the two types of bath is similar. They are both hot and they make you perspire profusely, so that the skin is left completely free of dirt.

The sauna is usually a small cabin-like, woodlined, cubicle with wide shelves on which you lie. They use dry heat, and are very hot, and you only spend ten minutes to half an hour at the most, in the sauna.

The Turkish bath is an altogether more leisurely affair and you spend at least 1–2 hours there. There may be several large rooms of varying heat, one or two hot steam rooms, and others which are less moist or less hot. You go from room to room, relaxing on deck chairs or on marble slabs, occasionally cooling down by swimming or splashing yourself with water. After you have relaxed, a masseur comes and gives you a shampooing. They rub you with a string or hemp glove to thoroughly clean the skin: great rolls of dirt and black skin are rubbed off. They then rub you with soap and massage you with the lather. Afterwards you're rinsed, sometimes even with a hose, the jets of cold water wakening you up! Then you go into another room (private or public) to recline and relax again.

I adore Turkish baths and visit them whenever I have the opportunity. They are generally so grandiose and beautiful that it is just like going back in time. You can almost imagine that you are an eastern princess in some exotic land.

After a Turkish Bath you emerge a new person, shining with cleanliness and totally refreshed and rejuvenated. It's as though you've just been on a long holiday – not just relaxing for a couple of hours.

Body scrubs

Elsewhere I've told you about scrubbing the body with your own string glove (see page 69), but it's appropriate after all the cleanliness induced by my description of a Turkish bath to mention a few more points here.

Oatmeal, gramflour or wheat flour can all be used. Simply mix the flour with milk and rub yourself with the mixture. One girl from Hyderabad, who used to use a well-known brand of cosmetics, found that in the winter her skin became very dry and patchy. She remembered that her grandmother used to wash with gramflour and so she started to use it herself. Within a week her skin had improved and so now she always uses it. Her grandmother also used to massage her body with a paste of gramflour and cream. This scrubbed the dirt off the skin and then she used handfuls of the dry flour to rub off the cream. Sometimes she added salt to the mixture as this is said to deter hair growth. This scrubbing of the skin keeps it smooth, supple, soft and shiny.

In India I used 'Khali', another mixture which is used as a body and face scrub. This is a mixture of crushed ground sesame seeds and jasmin flowers. This beautifully aromatic flour forms the basis of *'ubtan'* with which brides are massaged. This is a marvellous idea; ten days before the wedding the future bride is massaged each day with a paste made from this 'ubtan' and jasmin oil. In this way her skin becomes smooth as satin and delicately impregnated with jasmin oil. What could be more sophisticated or luxurious?

We could easily copy this, and try massaging ourselves (or a friend) with fine oatmeal (or gramflour) mixed into a paste with jasmin oil. It's worth trying because it really does leave one's skin feeling absolutely wonderful.

Week three

Don't forget

Every day
- (i)   Your daily exercises
- (ii) Your face cleaning, toning and creaming
- (iii) Your body washing, scrubbing and oiling

Once a week
- (i)   Your face and body massage
- (ii) Your hair conditioning and washing
- (iii) Your manicure and pedicure

This is the last week of your *Three-week health kick*, and you should literally be bouncing with health and vitality. Now you need concentrate on nothing but yourself and your body beautiful.

Sleep

One of the greatest of beautifiers, sleep regenerates our body and nerves and rejuvenates our faces. The body needs sleep – without it you become tense and nervous; indeed after ten days without sleep you can have hallucinations and even run the risk of death. Adults need between 6–8 hours' sleep. The body is rather like a battery, and in sleep charges up with energy. This charging happens during the first 6 hours of sleep (in fact, the energy starts to slip away again after 8–9 hours). You must have noticed sometimes that if you sleep too long, you wake up feeling tired. So you really don't need any longer than 8 hours.

I love sleeping and am always longing to go to sleep, and catch up on all those missing hours. But I recently read that we can't catch up on sleep. Sleep cannot be stored, and so it does us no good to go to bed really early the night after a late night. We cannot recapture the sleep we lost or store any for tomorrow. But even if this is true we can at least try and get our 8 hours that night.

There are three levels of sleep – shallow, deep and paradoxical. In the deep level, the body replaces dead cells and the body and the brain are completely relaxed. Dreams occur during paradoxical sleep. If you watch someone sleeping and see their eyelids moving (rapid eye movements) then they are at the paradoxical stage of sleep. It is now widely believed that dreaming is tremendously important. It is the time when the brain is sorting out all the information it has gained during the day, and without this paradoxical dreaming sleep, you become nervous, tired and depressed.

One of the most frustrating things in the world is not being able to sleep, but continued use of sleeping pills does not seem to be a very safe solution to the problem. Sleeping pills upset the pattern of sleep and reduce the amount of paradoxical sleep. That is one of the reasons why people who take a lot of sleeping pills often feel nervous and irritable, as though they have not slept properly. Another reason against continued usage of sleeping pills is that they can be addictive, until more and more, stronger and stronger, pills are needed. I've noticed that people who take sleeping pills are often very groggy in the mornings – the effect of all that drugged sleep. So try not to over-use sleeping pills – take them only as a last resort.

Instead, try taking calcium. Calcium is a natural tranquillizer and works wonders in helping you sleep. Before going to bed, prepare yourself a cup of hot milk – I know it is old-fashioned, but it is yet another of those old wives' tales which actually work (milk, of course, contains lots of calcium). Settle down in bed, drink your warm milk and take two calcium lactate tablets. If you are not asleep in an hour take another and so on until you fall asleep. With the soothing effect of the milk and calcium you should be asleep in no time. Several friends swear by this remedy.

The commonest reason for insomnia is that the insomniacs *believe* that they can't sleep, and this causes anxiety which in its turn causes sleeplessness (a vicious circle). So before even attempting to go to bed you need to relax. Try some of the relaxing exercises on page 155. If you go to bed feeling pleasantly relaxed you should be able to sleep. Again, exercise comes in here: a certain amount of exercise, preferably in the open air, helps to make one comfortably tired in both body and mind. Obvious stimulants such as coffee and alcohol and heavy food do not help in the search for lots of lovely sleep. As well as the hot milk and calcium remedy, try drinking a soothing herb tea – lime or chamomile are both renowned for their soothing effect.

If that still doesn't work, just try not to get worried about it. Maybe you don't actually need very much sleep. Get up and read, or write, then try doing the relaxing exercises and then maybe you'll have better luck.

'The famous physician Galen (AD 400) was in the habit of taking lettuce spiced with curry every night because it was thought to be a mild hypnotic. Galen used to say "These are my nights of sleep and more sleep".'

from *The General Principles of Avicenna's Canon of Medicine*

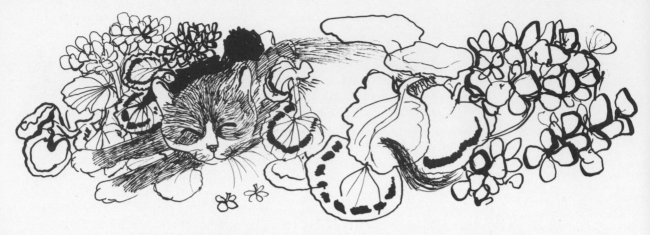

Cat napping

This is a marvellous way of catching up on sleep. Its efficacy lies in your ability to thoroughly relax (see page 156). These little naps throughout the day or evening can cut your need for night sleep by half. So learn to relax and have a cat nap. What a love life cats have, being stroked and having cat naps!

Beauty sleep

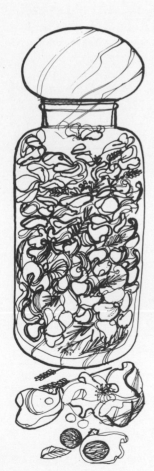

You must all have heard the saying that you need your beauty sleep – but I only recently discovered exactly why this was so important to the skin. As you know the skin is constantly repairing itself. The cells multiply by division rather like a brick building, and this activity is known as *mitosis*. But this process of mitosis is inhibited by chalone, a chemical which is reinforced by adrenalin. Adrenalin is needed to keep us active and energetic and so obviously the amount of adrenalin in our systems is greatest during the day. But when we sleep the adrenalin diminishes and so this cell division (mitosis) can then work more efficiently – and we wake up after a good night's sleep with a beautifully smooth, healthy, glowing skin.

When I learnt this it explained so many skin problems to me. For instance, hyper-nervous and tense people, and those going through periods of great stress, frequently suffer from bad skin. I presume that all the adrenalin they are producing reinforces the chalone and causes this poor skin condition.

As I mention in the exercise section, adrenalin needs to be used up not only for a feeling of well-being but also, as we now find out, for the skin. And so, if you tend to suffer from a bad skin it might help if you did more exercise. Try going out for a walk every day and sleep as much as possible. Remember exercise and sleep (and diet) are the bases of health.

Herb pillows and pot pourri

If you have difficulty in sleeping why not try a herb pillow? These were extremely popular amongst Victorians who used them to soothe their nerves and induce a refreshing sleep. They can be equally useful today, and insomniacs can frequently be induced to sleep with the help of a little herb pillow. The most common ingredient in these pillows is hops which are said to have an extremely soporific effect.

Nothing could be easier to make. Simply make a little cotton bag in the size you require and fill it with herbs. It's advisable to make a little slip cover for it so that it can be washed – use any pretty remnant or piece of old lace. These old-fashioned pillows take only a few minutes (about 15) to make and they are so pretty and useful. Scatter them around with the other cushions on your chair and they will smell beautiful. Sleep on them or give them away as presents – they are marvellous.

The Dragon Empress slept on pillows filled with rose petals and tea leaves so that the aroma filled the room and soothed her to sleep.

Use dried herbs and flowers to fill your cushions with – either fill them with pot pourri, or any mixture that you like – or have available. Here are some suggestions:

1. Hops, lavender, lemon verbena, sage, mint.
2. Rose petals, lavender, thyme and rose geranium, marjoram.
3. Rose petals, rosemary, lavender, jasmin, bergamot, lemon balm.

While you are making herb pillows you could also make some little herb sachets to hang in your cupboard and put amongst your clothes. Lavender was always used for this (lavender bags) but you can use anything aromatic. It's lovely and feels so luxurious opening drawers that smell beautiful.

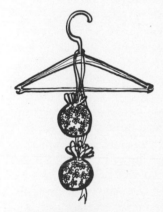

POT POURRI

3 cups dried rose petals
1 cup dried lavender
4 teaspoons coarse salt

2 tablespoons powdered
    orris root
1 teaspoon cinnamon
½ teaspoon nutmeg
½ teaspoon allspice
½ teaspoon ground cloves
¼ cup dried lemon balm
    (optional)
2 tablespoons rosemary
    (optional)
½ teaspoon anise seeds
    (optional)
¼ cup ground orange peel
    (optional)

As you must be looking and feeling so good by now, you might also want your home to look and smell good – so here is a recipe for Pot Pourri. You don't need hundreds of dried flowers and herbs – just one large bunch of roses and some lavender. When you have enjoyed the roses, instead of throwing them out take the petals off and dry them – just put them in the sun or lay them out in the airing cupboard.

Mix the petals, lavender and salt together in a large wide-necked jar and then seal the jar. After twelve hours add in all the spices and herbs. Mix everything together and there you are – you have made a marvellously fragrant mixture.

To make this smell even stronger I always add in a few drops of essential oil – ½ teaspoon rose oil, ¼ teaspoon jasmin oil, 10 drops bergamot oil.

There are many, many ways of making Pot Pourri – it is simply a question of putting any fragrant herbs and dried flowers together. Just mix anything that you have available and make your own personal Pot Pourri.

'We use the Orris root because it has the power of strengthening the other scents. It can also be put in the rinsing water to make clothes smell fresh. In 1480 it is mentioned in the wardrobe accounts of Edward IV where it was mixed with anise as a perfume for the linen.'

The Complete Herbal, M. Grieves

Stress, tension and depression

At some time all of us experience tension, anxiety, stress and depression. This may come about after a particularly irritating day, a long illness; or it might slowly creep up for no apparent reason. If our recuperative powers are good, with luck – and a little extra pampering, and rest and lots of sleep – we quickly recover. But for some, these states of stress are not so easily dispelled and tranquillizing pills are prescribed. With the ever-increasing pace of life the taking of pills is high and growing each year. *The Times* of April 5 1978 notes that 300 million doses of barbiturates were prescribed in 1976 (taken on a short-term basis they're extremely useful, but I don't believe they're a long-term solution).

To try and abolish stress would be impossible. Instead we need to learn to live with it and to try and overcome it. Primarily we need to find ways to release this tension and we need to learn to relax.

As Mennel the famous physiotherapist wrote in the 1930's, 'The advice to "pull yourself together" is really the worst that can be offered. Many patients owe their downfall to this mistaken sense of duty which has impelled them to "pull themselves together" instead of giving in and resting.' He found, as I have since, that massage can help relieve a feeling of anxiety and that it can help relax someone completely.

The massage should be of the gentlest type possible, using the softest stroking movements. This sets up a reflex action by relaxing the superficial skin and nerves, and gradually relaxes the whole body. (See the *Feather touch* on page 95.) In India this form of massage is known as '*kiri*' and is used to soothe and relax. Again, all the movements are soft, smooth, rhythmic and soporific. Next time anyone you know is feeling especially tense or tired do try it – or persuade someone to do it for you.

A very simple way of releasing tension is to roll on the floor. Lie on the floor and roll from one side of the room to the other. This rolling rids you of static electricity and has the most remarkably relaxing effect. The Mongols used this technique to relax themselves after a long day in the saddle.

Another method of relaxation is this exercise from Turkey called '*Takhfif*' – the 'lightness'. This exercise was for many centuries a closely guarded secret of the Imperial Ottomans. Lie down and direct your thoughts to your limbs. Starting with your right foot. Relax your toes and foot, imagine that they are weightless. Then repeat the same process of relaxation with your right leg, the right side of your body and up to the shoulder. Then do the same with your right hand, fingers first, and again to the shoulder, neck and head.

Repeat in the same manner up the left side. Then imagine that there is a soft current of ease and relaxation passing through your whole body, in the same succession, smoothly and continuously. It has a marvellous lightening effect.

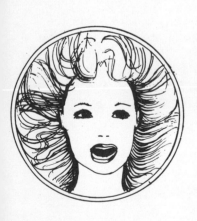

Another quick tension reliever is to open your mouth as wide as possible. It sounds crazy but if you try it you will find that it works. A friend who lived in Japan told me that his acupuncture doctor used to make him open his mouth wide at intervals throughout his treatments

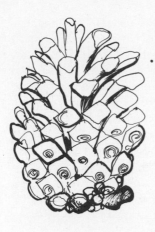

because he was so tense. I think that it's great fun to discover these marvellous, zany, but effective cures. This one can be explained by the fact that in the lower cheek between the ear and the mouth there is a large nerve centre where a tremendous amount of tension accumulates. By opening the mouth wide the muscles are stretched and the tension is released.

In an ancient Afghan manuscript it is recommended that Jalaghoza nuts (pine kernels) are eaten as a cure for depression. About $\frac{1}{4}$ oz/7–8 g are to be eaten once a day for several days. I was told that this would have a slightly stimulating effect because they contain minute amounts of strychnine which is a stimulant.

Hands and feet

And now for something completely different. Check your hands and feet. They should be smooth and soft by now, with all the care that I hope you are lavishing on them. Use a pumice stone to remove any hard, horny skin from the soles of your feet, but if they still need some help try this hand and foot cleanser.

1 oz/25 g ground almonds
¼ pint/150 ml milk
1 egg yolk
1 teaspoon oil
2 drops lemon oil

Bring the almonds and milk to the boil and remove from the heat. Stir in the egg yolk, and then put it back on the heat. Keep stirring until the mixture thickens. Then add the oils and remove from the heat.

Rub this ensuing paste into the skin until it begins to dry. Always do this over the bath or a sink because it will suddenly start to peel off great rolls of black muck. This looks quite revolting but is the most fantastic cleanser, really getting rid of ingrained dirt and callouses. Don't only use it on your feet and hands – elbows, knees and even necks and faces can all benefit from a good scrub. If you are feeling very keen you could massage the whole of your body with it. After rubbing with this paste the skin is left looking beautifully clean and feeling incredibly smooth and soft.

Smelly feet

Just in case anyone you know suffers from 'smelly feet' I would like to pass on this remedy that a woman from Stafford kindly sent to me. She told me that her sister's husband suffered so badly from this complaint that she had difficulty in washing his socks. Someone told him to soak his feet for an hour in hot water in which ivy leaves had been boiled. He followed this advice, and soaked his feet several days in succession. The remedy was a complete success and he never again suffered from perspiration of the feet.

Scent

'Scents are surer than sounds to make your heart strings crack.' Rudyard Kipling

You should be looking and feeling marvellous by now and applying scent just adds the finishing touch. Using your favourite perfume is one of the best ways to make you feel instantly more attractive. There are simply hundreds from which to choose, ranging from fresh and light to heavy, sexy or exotic, and it is simply a question of finding one to suit the mood of the moment.

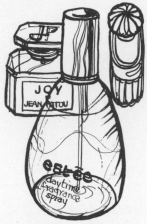

Every scent is slightly different on different individuals – just because it smells good on someone else does not necessarily mean it will suit you. To find out if a perfume suits you, you must first try it by wearing it. Apply some on your wrist, give it time to react to the heat of your body and then smell it in about 15 minutes. Don't try and test several perfumes on the same day because your nose will become confused. Just test one at a time until you find what you want.

There are fashions in perfume as there are in everything else. Among the ancient Greeks the scents of violets and other similar flowers were very popular, and amongst the upper classes the fainter the scent was the better. Later when the heavier scents were imported from the East, these became fashionable. The same applied in the Victorian era, as we can see by this quote on perfume from Foulsham's *Enquire Within*:

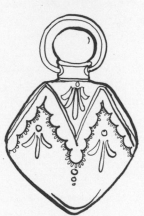

'The lady of breeding is known by her perfumes. Scent should never be used in such a way as to be immediately obvious; the wise woman applies just sufficient of a good perfume to leave an indefinite suggestion, rather than a positive assertion, of its presence. Eau-de-cologne, lavender and Parma Violets, or, in fact, any of the old-fashioned perfumes are rarely out of place, but the more exotic preparations are apt to be in rather questionable taste, and should only be indulged in with caution.'

Although nowadays there is no question of exotic scents being in bad taste, they can be rather overpowering if used too lavishly. Most perfumes have only a four-hour life span, as they evaporate with body heat, and so it is better to reapply a little scent frequently rather than smother yourself only once. Put the scent anywhere you tend to perspire: the temples, behind the earlobes, the wrists, behind the knees and at the ankles. As Diogenes said 300 years before Christ: 'When you annoint your head with perfume it flies into the air and only the birds obtain any benefit. But when applied to the legs and feet, the scents envelop the whole body and gradually ascend the nose.'

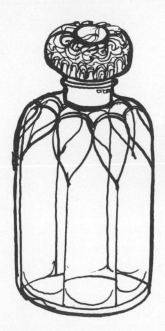

A friend puts a small piece of cotton wool soaked in perfume between her breasts (in her bra), and this is a very good way of applying perfume. The scent seems to last longer on the cotton wool than when applied straight to the skin. The idea of applying perfume in this way is very ancient. In King Solomon's time myrrh was extremely popular and the women would put a small cotton bag containing myrrh and sweet smelling herbs between their breasts under their clothes. The heat of the body released the scent so that it could be enjoyed by all – the wearer and those near by. *The Song of Solomon* records 'A bundle of myrrh is my well-beloved unto me; he shall lie all night betwixt my breasts', and in Robert Graves' version of the *Song of Songs*: 'Your lips, my love, are like honeycomb, honey and milk flow from under your tongue and your garments breathe incense.'

Although myrrh is now rarely used by itself as a perfume it is still greatly used in medicine and as a fixative for perfumes, as are gum-arabic (a gum from one of the acacia trees) and musk. Musk was tremendously popular amongst the early Arabs. They so loved the smell that when building they would mix musk with the mortar, and

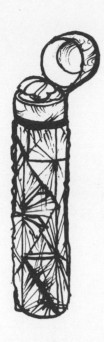

in the Kontbia mosque at Marrakesh in Morocco one can still smell its fragrance. Musk is obtained from the male musk deer of Central Asia. Chemists have succeeded in manufacturing a synthetic equivalent but it doesn't have the same lasting power. It is however infinitely cheaper (real musk being more costly than gold!), and in fact a great number of the essential oils available to us are synthetic because the natural oils are *so* expensive.

Rose oil has always been greatly prized and is still one of the most commonly used and popular perfumes. Most quality perfumes contain either rose oil, or jasmin, to add smoothness and depth to the perfume.

One last word about scent – don't always wait for perfumes to be given to you. I know the initial outlay may seem high but they give so much pleasure and last such a long time that they are a worthwhile investment. So, go on and treat yourself to your favourite perfume.

Aromatic oils

Aromatic oils are very useful and tremendously easy to make. They can be used to massage with, can be used in the bath, put into your creams, and even poured on your salads to make them taste more exotic. You can use any fragrant herbs or flowers, either by themselves or in a mixture: bay, tarragon, lavender and rosemary, basil, thyme, or rose and jasmin – the possibilities are endless.

Crush two tablespoons of the herbs or flowers and put them into a half pint/300 ml bottle, three quarters fill this with almond or sunflower oil and add one tablespoon vodka (or white wine vinegar). Cork the bottle and place it in strong sunlight. Shake the bottle a couple of times a day. After about ten days strain the oil and repeat the process with fresh herbs. Carry on repeating the process until the oil smells strong enough for you.

If there is no strong sunlight, put the bottle in a double boiler and gently heat the oil (keeping the water just below boiling point) for an hour every day. Do this every day for a week and then strain and repeat until the oil smells strongly aromatic.

Another way of making this oil is to put a layer of cotton wool at the bottom of the jar, saturate it with almond oil, then put in an inch thick layer of flowers or herbs, cover them with another layer of impregnated cotton wool. Carry on making layers of cotton wool and flowers until the jar is full. Pack it tightly, then seal it well and put in a warm, dark place for ten days. Replace the flowers or herbs with fresh ones and repeat the process. When the oil smells strong enough, squeeze the oil from the cotton wool and enjoy using your own oil.

These aromatic oils are lovely, so do make some, and experiment with all the different combinations.

The last word on exercise

Are you still doing at least 5 minutes of exercise every day?

If you find that you are getting slack about doing your exercises turn back to the exercise section and refresh your memory – or if you really cannot find those few minutes at least do this one, easy but *most effective* exercise, I learnt it from a girl friend who has done it religiously every day for the last ten years, she has a marvellous figure which she attributes to this.

STRETCH

Stand with your feet apart and reach up towards the ceiling. Or do it in the doorway and try and reach the top of the doorway. Stretch up – first one arm and then the other. Stretch five times on each side.

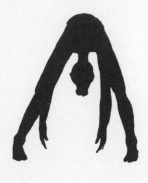

FLOP

Breathing out, bend down, aiming to touch the floor. Bounce down towards the floor five times.

STRETCH

At the bottom of your bounce, stretch through your legs and aim to touch the floor behind you. Then bring your arms up until they are in a parallel line to the floor, do not lean backwards. Your body and waist should be at a 90° angle. In this position again bounce ten times. This is only a small movement, and makes you use the muscles in the small of the back.

Repeat this whole exercise a couple of times. It is marvellous, really stretching you and making you feel wide awake.

Finish by flopping your head down as though you were a rag doll. Stay in that lovely relaxed position for about a minute. All the blood will rush to your head (not quite as effective as the head stand but still very good).

Shiatsu

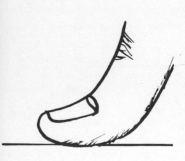

The word *shiatsu* is made up of two Japanese characters: *shi* – finger, and *atsu* – pressure, and that is exactly what it is – finger pressure.

Shiatsu, as it is practised today, was evolved about 50 years ago in Japan. It is derived from the primitive action of rubbing a painful area, and also, like acupuncture, on the belief that there are key points on the body meridians down which energy is said to flow. Instead of inserting needles in the body at these main points, one applies pressure. These pressures are thought to unblock a flow of energy.

Shiatsu is essentially a preventative medicine. Pressures applied to key points accelerate the circulation and release tension. They relieve fatigue, headaches, aching shoulders and generally make one feel healthier.

In Japan, qualified Shiatsu practitioners treat illnesses, but this is obviously a job for the professionals. No one knows exactly why these pressures have an effect on the body, but they appear to give beneficial results so it is certainly worth trying.

These pressures are usually performed with the thumbs, although the fingers and palms can also be used. Press down with the ball of the thumb. Be careful not to use the tip as that makes the pressure uncomfortable, and your nails, however short, will gouge the skin. My shiatsu teacher's thumbs went back almost at right angles. Pressure from the ball of the thumb is softer as the fat there cushions the pressure, and however firm it is, it will not be painful. The pressure should be even and vary in intensity from 5 to 15 pounds, and the duration is between 3 to 7 seconds.

Practise this pressure by pushing down on a pair of bathroom scales. You will find that with the heavy pressures you need to use the weight of your body. Lean in towards your friend to ensure that your pressure is even – by using your body it will also prevent your arms from becoming tired.

At some of these pressure points there are clusters of nerves, and pressure applied there can be very painful. It is important, however, to stimulate these areas, so don't leave them out: just press gently at first, until either you, or your partner, can take more pressures.

Anyone can perform simple shiatsu treatments. This is one form of massage it is easy to give to yourself as you can reach most of the points without too much of a strain.

Although there are over 600 shiatsu points, I have only shown the key points in the diagrams. Try them all and see which ones you find the most beneficial. Everyone has different needs.

You can give a treatment composed entirely of shiatsu, or you can incorporate some of the pressures into your massages. My assistants and I find shiatsu incredibly useful. Knowing the shiatsu points, it has become second nature to us to blend the pressures into our massage. We are able to cure clients of their aches and pains and generally make them feel better. So do try giving yourself, or a friend, a treatment and hopefully it will relieve your tensions, increase your vitality and give you a wonderful feeling of well-being.

Although my diagrams might make you think that it is difficult to find such small precise points on the body, it is far easier than it looks. It is surprising how often there are little indentations to help you find the correct spot. So use your intuition, your eyes and your fingers to feel for them – also ask your friend, who will be able to tell you when you are on the correct place.

Never do this, or any other massage, to anyone who has recently had a slipped disc, or any chronic back problems. When in doubt, always check with a doctor.

THE BACK OF THE BODY

The shoulders, neck and back

1. Apply pressures up the neck on either side of the spine. A key point is at the base of the skull where there is an actual indentation. Press hard and work out towards the ears, on the edge of the skull, working simultaneously on both sides. These pressures not only relax the patient but relieve sinus congestion and headaches.

2. Press hard on the top of the shoulder, where as you press you will feel a well between the shoulder and the collar-bone. This energy point is marvellous for relieving stiff shoulders and general tension in that area.

3.   Press at the centre of the shoulder blade. This relieves pain in the upper back and arms.

4.   There are points running on either side of the entire length of the spine. Using your thumbs work on both sides simultaneously. There is a major point at waist level, which helps to relax the whole back.

5.   Apply pressure in the little indentations (dimples) of the lower back and down that kindly placed triangle to the coccyx. This relieves tension in the lower back, period pains, and I have even helped ease the stiffness caused by lumbago.

6.   Apply pressure to the points on the outer hip, in the middle of the buttock and actually under the crease of the bottom. The point in the centre of each buttock might be rather painful as it is a nerve centre, but is an important point for relieving tension. Remember that the pain doesn't last and in fact is actually relieving tension – a client calls this 'grateful hurt'.

All these points are important ones for relieving tension of the hips and lower back. Some people get their tension in their bottoms and so this obviously helps them.

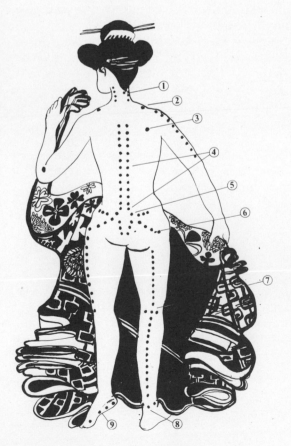
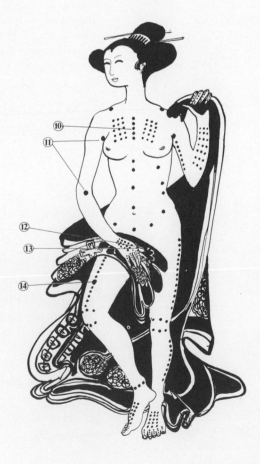

Leg and foot

7.   There is a meridian of points running the length of the back for the leg. Use your thumbs for pressure on this line. Many sportsmen suffer from cramp and tight muscles and this pressure helps. There is a major point behind the centre of the knee, and pressure here has a tremendously relaxing effect, and also calms any stomach pain.

8.   On the Achilles tendon there is another major point. Pressure here relieves pain in the lower back and the nagging stomach ache that some women suffer during menstruation. Apply pressure actually on the tendon, and in the recesses on either side.

9.   A major energy point is located in the centre of the sole of the foot – this is known as the 'fountain of energy' and it really seems to live up to its name. (See page 143 for more information on feet.)

THE FRONT OF THE BODY

Chest, arm and hand

10.   These pressures across the chest help anyone who suffers from chest problems, asthma or bronchial conditions and anyone who suffers from liver problems.

11.   There is a point right in the centre of the arm pit. Apply pressure here, and at the point on the inside of the elbow, and then all the way down the meridian on the inside of the forearm. These points are excellent for anyone with tired arms – pianists, knitters, gardeners, writers, etc.

12.   On the hand in between the thumb and forefinger there is a major point, and another in the centre of the palm (13). Both of these are energy points that can envigorate splendidly when you are tired. It is very easy to press your own hands, so you can try it yourself.

14.   This point relates to the knee and so if you suffer from stiff knees, press here for relief.

HEAD AND FACE

Pressures on the face and head are extremely relaxing, increasing circulation to the brain and making one instantly feel better and more clear-headed. Even before I researched and learnt shiatsu, I had discovered the importance of these points. I had always applied pressure on these very same positions and it became obvious to me that my clients found them incredibly relaxing.

I was tempted to describe these pressure points in the section on face massage but decided that as they are the very ones used in shiatsu they would be best described here – otherwise I'd be repeating myself and would bore you. But really do try and learn these points and use them. You will be amazed at their remarkable effect. They are quick and easy to do anywhere – on suffering friends, or even on yourself.

Hangover cure (1)
I have found that if a client is suffering from a hangover and I apply pressure to the 'third eye' and up in a straight line to the back of the head, the symptoms very soon diminish and often miraculously disappear!

Headache cure (1, 2, 3, 6)
Any one of the points will be beneficial, and your best guide for which is the *most* effective, will be your friend.

Cold and sinus relief (2, 5, 6)
Apply pressure at the points around the ears and at the base of the skull. These work almost instantly, unblocking the sinuses and helping to clear up colds.

General tension and aching eyes (4, 6, 7)
Again, let your friend be your guide.

Face
On the face the pressure is obviously not as hard as on the head and you usually use the tips of the fingers and not the thumbs.

When the point under the eyebrow is pressed some clients have told me that they feel fantastic, as though their head is suffused with colour.

All these points are incredibly easy to incorporate into the facial massage (see page 108), simply by applying extra pressure during any movement.

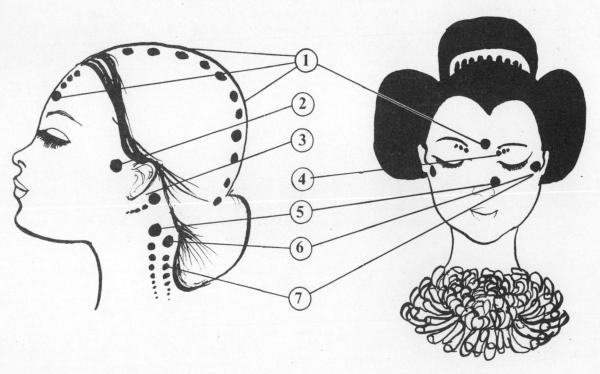

Zone therapy and Reflexology

Zone therapy and reflexology, like shiatsu (see page 138), is also a type of pressure-point massage related to the body meridians, but applied mainly to the feet.

Different areas of the foot are thought to relate to all the parts of the body, and by applying pressure to the feet you can treat the whole body. Again, no one really knows why this, or any other similar technique, works, and there have been no explanations to satisfy Western scientists. But there definitely is a correlation, and some people find the treatment tremendously successful. Headaches, back-aches, and sinus problems can all be helped – and at the very least most people enjoy having their feet massaged. I am amazed at the number of people who apparently bribe their children with extra pocket money to rub their feet!

Here are simple diagrams of the points and the areas they relate to – and so it is up to you to experiment on either yourself or a friend.

Right foot   Left foot

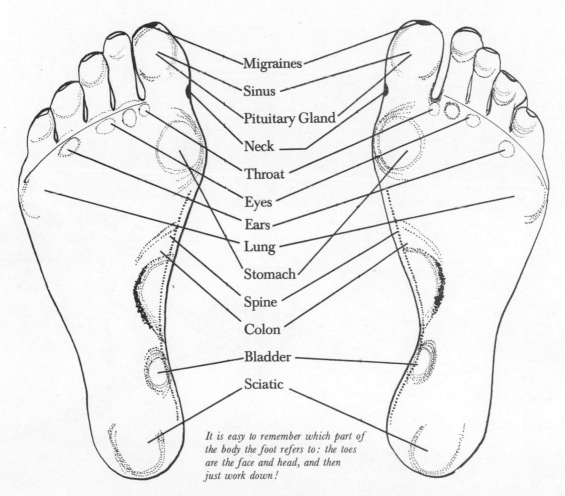

Migraines
Sinus
Pituitary Gland
Neck
Throat
Eyes
Ears
Lung
Stomach
Spine
Colon
Bladder
Sciatic

It is easy to remember which part of the body the foot refers to: the toes are the face and head, and then just work down!

'One day the Emperor Hadrian saw a veteran soldier rubbing himself against the marble wall at the Roman public baths and asked him why he did so. The veteran answered that he was too poor to have a slave rub him and this was the best substitute he could find, wherepon the Emperor got him two slaves and enough money to maintain them. A few days later several old men rubbed themselves against the wall in the Emperor's presence hoping for similar good fortune, but the shrewd Hadrian, perceiving their object, ordered them to rub one another.'

Graham, *A Treatise on Massage*, 1902

'Women are most fascinating between the ages of 35 and 40 after they have won a few races and know how to pace themselves. Since few women ever pass 40, maximum fascination can continue indefinitely.'

Christian Dior (in *Collier's*, 1955)

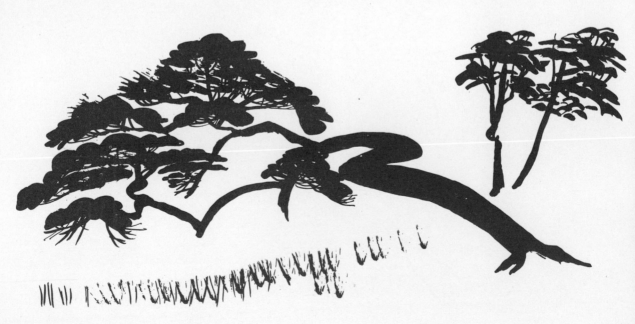

Exercise

As I write the word 'exercise' I can practically feel you giving a mental groan and 'switching off', all ready to skip the whole of this chapter. Please don't.

Why we should exercise

The main reason for exercising is that it makes you feel and look so much healthier, and gives you a feeling of well-being.

By stimulating the action of your heart and lungs, you help prevent heart attacks, your whole body works more efficiently, and there is increased oxidation to the body cells. Your circulation is stimulated and your skin improved.

In the course of a busy day your body releases large amounts of adrenalin which goes into the bloodstream. This enables you to keep going and cope with the stresses and dramas of the day; but if the adrenalin is not completely utilized by physical activity, it is stored. And it is this which can affect your emotions, making you feel exhausted or depressed. Exercise, of any sort, metabolizes this adrenalin and so that is why, when you are exhausted after work, a few minutes of exercise would do more to revitalize you and increase your serenity than any cocktail. Don't believe or disbelieve me – try it.

Exercise can also be invaluable in preventing backache. I know many people who suffer from aching backs, and they tell me that if they do their exercises, the aches either greatly diminish or disappear completely. By improving your muscle tone through exercise, your posture should also automatically improve and one woman told me that she was actually two inches taller since she had taken up exercising!

Why we don't exercise

The idea of exercise so often conjures up bleak visions of exhausting work-outs, hearty physical jerks, or jogging around the block on a cold day. With this image it is hardly surprising that you hate the thought of exercises. But they do not have to be like that – exercising can be easy and enjoyable.

First of all, don't aim too high. Set your standards low. If you have never done any regular exercise before, start by doing a few of those lovely, relaxing, stretching exercises – you will find them so enjoyable that you will soon be doing more happily. If you aim too high, and try to do too much at first, you are bound to get bored, disheartened and give up trying. Instead do only a few; then slowly, as you become fitter, you will automatically do more because you *want* to, not because you have to.

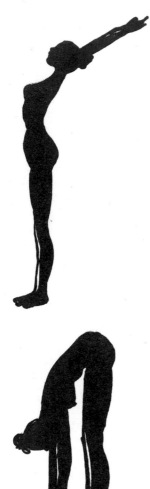

You can always find time for something that you enjoy – so make exercises as enjoyable as possible. Find your own pace. Don't expect miracles. Slowly and surely you will become fitter and feel healthier.

If one day you really do not want to do your exercises – skip them. It doesn't matter, you can always do them tomorrow. Do not feel (as some people do) that if you miss one day, you have ruined everything, and so may as well give up altogether.

You can start exercising at any age, if you go at your own tempo. We know that as we get older we generally become less fit. I don't think that this is an inevitable result of age, but because we become more sedentary. Substitute activity for inactivity. A little regular exercise helps you to live longer, and makes you feel better and younger.

Energy makes energy – so let's get exercising!

I have divided these exercises into two sections which I have called *Warmers* and *Shapers*, but when going through them I realized that a lot of the warmers were very important shapers. My idea was that you could do the standing exercises (warmers) early every morning before starting your work – and the floor exercises (shapers) in the evening, or whenever you had more time. The standing exercises constitute the *minimum* programme and should be done every single day. The floor exercises are for when you are having a blitz on yourself.

If you only have a couple of minutes each day, then do some of the stretching exercises from the selection of warmers. They are incredibly easy to do. They are enjoyable and only need take as little as five minutes. I find that if I plan to do only a five-minute session, I do manage to squeeze it in every day; but once I think it is going to take me ten to fifteen minutes, up comes that psychological block and I won't do any at all. However, the funny thing is that if you think you can only do five minutes, it very often turns into ten or fifteen minutes! In fact, I met a woman who said she started out doing only five or ten minutes a day (to music) but became so enthusiastic, and felt so much healthier, that she now does nearly an hour's work-out every weekday.

The second section is for such enthusiasm – when you have mastered the first section – and they too are very, very easy. You will want (I hope) to go on to do more – and that is what these floor exercises (shapers) are for.

I have spent a long time choosing and working out the sequence of the exercises, so that they flow easily from one to another. This is because I really do want you not only to try them once, but to keep doing them each day.

These exercises are my own and my clients' favourites, the ones we have found the most effective and enjoyable. We found that if we did them all to music, they were less of a chore and much more fun to do; so put on your favourite music and get moving. The exercises are designed to make your body feel expanded, open and full of life; to make you feel invigorated, in a good mood, and able to face the world.

I have explained the exercises very fully to ensure that you learn them correctly and get the most benefit out of them. So the first time you do them, it might take you an hour, reading my descriptions and then trying them out. But as soon as you know them, which doesn't take long at all, you can then use my quick check list and romp through them all in no time at all. (I have even managed to do all the warmers in five minutes in someone's loo!)

It is worth taking a little time to learn how to make your body feel good – after all, you take tennis, swimming, or cooking lessons. You make sure that your car is in good running order by having it regularly serviced; and you're not surprised if it breaks down, or even falls to pieces, if you don't. But what do you do for your poor old neglected body?

Here is the quick check list:

Quick check list

Warmers – standing exercises
1. Deep breathing
2. Stretching
3. Controlled flop
4. Knee bends
5. Side bends
6. Catherine wheel
7. Torso twisting
8. Leg swinging
9. Bust and chest
10. Running or dancing on the spot
11. Shaking
12. Shoulder rolling
13. Head rolling

Shapers – floor exercises
1. Pelvic tilt
2. Sit-ups
3. Leg lifting
4. Hip rolling
5. Bicycling in the air
6. Side scissors
7. Backward scissors
8. The cobra
9. Forward roll
10. Shoulder stand

Warmers (standing exercises)

These are stretching and loosening exercises, and should all be done five to ten times, every day.

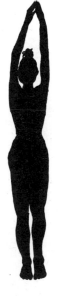

1. *Deep breathing*
(a)   Stand with your feet together and arms hanging down at your sides. As you breathe in, lift your arms out to the side and above your head. Breathing out, return to the starting position. It is a large circular movement. Breathe in and raise up, breathe out and down.

(b)   Nearly the same, but this time, as you breathe in, you swing your arms forward and up above your head, and raise yourself up onto your toes. Stretch as high as possible, breathing out as you return to the starting position.

2. *Stretching*
(a)   Reach up as high as you can with one arm, and then reach up with the other. Aim for the ceiling. As you do this stretching, be aware

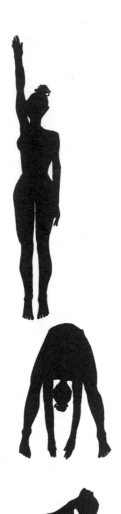

of your body. Your stomach should be held in, and buttock muscles contracted tightly. Reach up with one arm, stretch – and stretch, then with the other arm stretch – and stretch. Feel the pull down the side of your body. This is one of my favourite exercises, it is so easy and effective. One friend does this at least a hundred times each day, and attributes her marvellous figure to it. Do at *least* ten times.

3. *Controlled flop*
(a) Stand with your feet apart and your knees straight. Breathing out, you bend down from the waist, aiming to touch the floor, but with your back and arms relaxed. Bounce down towards the floor five times. Then breathing in, rise up, swinging your arms forward and up towards the ceiling. This is a relaxed floppy movement. Repeat five times.

(b) Same starting position. Bounce five times towards the floor and five times through your legs, aiming as far behind you as possible.
     Then bring your arms up until they are parallel to the floor. Do not lean back, but try and keep your legs perpendicular to the floor, so that your body is at a 90° angle. In this position bounce ten times. To do this bounce properly, you must keep your back and knees straight and hold yourself in at the stomach and buttocks. It is quite difficult at first. Bounce ten times and then return to the standing position and repeat the whole exercise.
     When you are doing this exercise correctly you will feel the effect all the way down the backs of your legs. It is also very good for exercising the lower back muscles. So, although difficult at first, this is a terrific exercise and worth your while to persevere with.
     When you have completed the exercise, relax your legs by shaking them.

(c) These are gentle back bends to balance the previous exercise. Stand straight with your feet slightly apart. Clasp your hands behind you, and bend back from the waist letting your head flop backwards. Then bounce backwards. As your head and back bounce, your hips will move forward a little. Keep your arms as relaxed as possible – there should be no strain attached to this easy exercise.

4. *Knee bends*
(a) Stand erect, feet apart, with toes pointing slightly outward and arms hanging loosely by your sides. Lower your body into a squatting position, keeping your heels flat on the floor for as long as possible, your knees pressing outward and your back and head in a straight line. Come up slowly, imagining a string pulling you up from the top of your head. Place your heels on the ground as soon as possible. You will undoubtedly feel this exercise in the tops of your thighs and if you are doing it correctly, with your knees well turned out, it exercises those problem inner-thigh muscles.

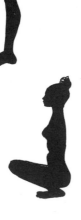

(b) Stand with your back straight, feet and knees together (that is the difficult bit). Rise up onto your toes and with your back still very straight, bounce down into the squatting position. Bounce up and down, up and down, staying on your toes all the time. This can either be done fast, when it improves your balance, or slowly, when it's good for your back and leg muscles.

(c)   After that energetic exercise, relax by standing as long as possible on one leg. Raise one knee up in front of you, keeping the other leg and back straight, balanced like a flamingo. Again this is marvellous for your legs. Hold that position for as long as possible, then balance on the other leg.

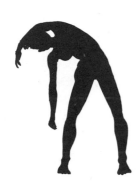

5.   *Side bends*
(a)   Feet apart, bend first to the right, then to the left, face forward, but be sure to keep the hips and bottom held firm. Do it rhythmically.

(b)   The same exercise, but this time you also use your arms. Bend first to the right with your left arm above your head (held as close to your ear as possible) and the right arm hanging down loosely, towards your knee. Three bends to the right, then bounce up, swinging your right arm up and your left arm goes down, bend three times to the left. Again your whole body must be in a straight line – don't allow either your stomach or bottom to stick out. This is especially good for the waist.

6.   *Catherine wheel*
(a)   Start with your feet apart, standing erect with your hands above your head. Swing the arms to the right, and then, flopping forward, swing down to brush the floor. Carry on up to the left and swing around behind you to complete a full circle. Try and remember to swing side, forward, side, back; side, forward, side, back. Do this lovely, large, circular movement three times to the right, and then at the bottom swing, reverse, and circle in the other direction. This exercise is bliss, without doubt my favourite. It stretches all the stomach and waist muscles and gives one such a feeling of freedom and well-being.

7.   *Torso twisting*
(a)   Stand erect, arms out to your side. Twist your torso from side to side, keeping your hips motionless and facing forward; twist, trying to look behind you, allowing your arms to swing freely, but always keeping them at shoulder level. It is an easy relaxed movement but try and reach as far behind you as you can. Good for the abdominal muscles, and will help you to have a strong back and flat stomach.

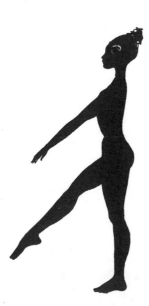

8.   *Leg swinging*
(a)   Stand erect, feet together, tummy and bottom pulled in. Swing your right leg, toes pointed, forward and back. If you find it easier, swing your arms as well; left arm forward when right leg is forward. If you find it difficult to keep your pelvis still, place the flat of one hand on your tummy and the other on your bottom, and *make* it stay still. Ten times with one leg and then the other.

(b)   Lift and bend the right leg and move it out to the right side. Swing the leg down, across and up to the left side, and return down, across the back to the right hand side, like a pendulum. Do this ten times each side. Of course, throughout this exercise your supporting leg must be straight, your tummy held in and your hips facing forward.

You may find it easier to do these exercises holding on to the back of a chair or the side of a table – but as you get fitter, dispense with these props and use your own muscles as support.

9. *Bust and chest*
(a)   Stand erect with elbows out, and place your palms together. While pressing the whole of your hands together circle them inwards towards your chest, and still maintaining full pressure slowly circle out. Try and repeat three times without slackening the pressure. Then relax and repeat. You can feel the interior muscles which support the bust contracting. This always reminds me of Thai dancing.

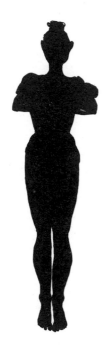

(b)   Standing erect, place the palms together at shoulder level. Press the whole of your hands firmly together. Hold for the count of four, relax the pressure, link fingers and try and pull your hands apart to the count of four. Push two, three, four, relax, link, pull two, three, four, relax. Repeat at least ten times.

(c)   Raise your arms to shoulder level and grasp each forearm. Push against your forearms and feel your pectoral muscle 'jump'. This is an exercise we all know and really should do.

In these chest exercises exert your muscles to their maximum. Push as hard as you can and remember to keep your elbows level with your shoulders. These exercises should be done every single day – there's no excuse. Do them while you wait for the kettle to boil. Try and do them at least fifty times a day. The results will make it worth that little bit of effort.

10.   *Running or dancing on the spot*
(a)   At first do this easily and gently, and, as you get fitter, you will be able to lift your knees higher and go faster. Doing this to music is great fun – honestly it is. I know you don't believe me so you had better try it and see. One girl I met started doing this two hundred times a day, and found that she enjoyed it so much that she now does two thousand!

Relax and breathe deeply.

11.   *Shaking*
(a)   Now shake out your limbs. Really shake out one arm, then the other and now the legs. It makes one feel rather like a rag doll. Try shaking in time to the music; it's a crazy feeling.

This shaking exercise was a favourite of a friend's grandmother who was still exercising at the age of eighty-four. She had such a good figure that all her family have followed her example and all of them exercise daily.

12.   *Shoulder rolling*
(a)   Stand erect, with your tummy and bottom pulled in. Rest your fingers on your shoulders and describe a large circle with your elbows. Remember to make a full circle by going forward, up, back and down.

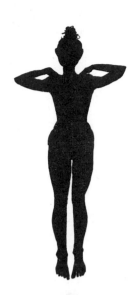

Five going forward then five backwards.

(b)   With your arms hanging loosely down by your sides, lift your shoulders up towards your ears. Then relax the muscles and drop them. Push them down even further. Lift, drop, push, lift, drop, push. Both shoulders together and then try one at a time.

(c)   Roll your right shoulder up and forward and then up and back to its normal position, then roll up and back and roll up to return to the starting position. Repeat with the left shoulder.

Do these exercises to music. Vary the routine; try moving both shoulders together forward and back, or move one shoulder forward as the other goes back and vice versa. You can get quite muddled if the music is fast, which makes it all the more fun.

These exercises are marvellous for round shoulders, and they're also the simplest way of relieving shoulder tension which is often the cause of headaches, particularly if you do a lot of desk work.

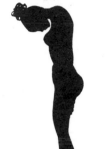

13.   *Head rolling*

(a)   Drop your head forward (feel the weight drop down). Pull it upright again and drop it backwards (feel those back muscles stretch). Forward, upright, back. Forward, upright, back.

(b)   Turn your head from side to side, trying to look at the wall behind you. Side, forward, side. Side, forward, side.

(c)   Drop your head to the side, trying to touch your shoulder with your ear – but without lifting your shoulders. Drop to the side, upright, and then to the other side.

(d)   Drop the head forward, and slowly circle it around and around. Five times going one way, and five times the other. Roll forward, side, back, side. This is a most important and relaxing exercise. It is lovely to do; feel all those muscles stretching; you can even feel the ones in the base of the spine being worked. It is miraculous for relieving tension, and making your head feel light and clear.

Now breathe deeply and relax and you have finished your standing exercises. It was quite fun, wasn't it?

I hope that this will have made you madly enthusiastic and energetic; if you are not dashing off to work you could do some of the floor (shaping-up) exercises (or you can leave them until this evening).

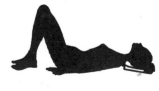

Shapers (floor exercises)

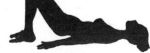

1.   *Pelvic tilt*

(a)   Lie on your back with your knees bent, feet on the floor and arms by your side. Contract your stomach, and you will find that your pelvis moves up and your back presses down into the floor. Hold that position for a second, and then roll the pelvis down and the back will arch off the ground. Roll your pelvis up and down, don't strain, just do it gently and rhythmically. This strengthens and improves the flexibility of the back and works those tummy muscles. (You can also do this exercise standing up by pressing your back against the wall.)

(b)   This exercise which I call the '*Triangle*' is a continuation of the last exercise. This time when you contract your stomach, you also contract your bottom and thigh muscles, and lift your body up until you make a triangle. Hold that position, and then by starting from the top of the spine, unroll each vertebra slowly one by one, until you have returned to the starting position.

2.   *Sit-ups*

(a)   Lie on the floor with legs straight. Lift your head and look at your flexed toes. Look at your toes again, this time lifting your shoulders up as well. Now try and lift your whole trunk, sit up and bend over towards your straight legs. As you breathe in, lift your arms and body up. Keep your legs straight, your tummy in, and your feet flexed. Go as far forward as possible with your head going down towards your knees. Unroll very slowly to the starting position.

The easiest way to do sit-ups is to start with your hands behind your head (some people like to hold a stick, a ruler is ideal). The swing of your arms going forward aids your stomach muscles to lift your body off the floor. And the exercise is made easier if you lodge your feet under something, a sofa or armchair, or get a friend to hold your feet down.

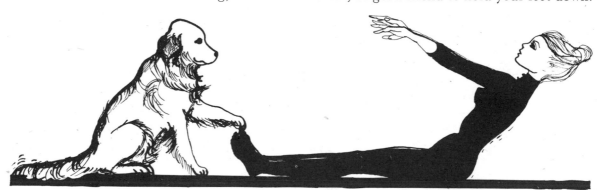

As your stomach muscles strengthen try doing sit-ups with your arms lying relaxed by your sides – but don't cheat and push yourself up with your elbows. Those with very strong abdominal muscles clasp their fingers behind their necks, but I find I must have my feet lodged to be able to lift up by even half an inch from this position. Athletes do hundreds of sit-ups on severely inclining boards (to make it harder) holding weights above their heads.

You should be able to work up to about fifty a day.

Do the whole exercise as slowly as possible; although it is more difficult done slowly, it gives you better control over your muscles. Go only as far as you can with comfort. Don't strain – if it hurts, stop; soon you will be doing it easily.

When I asked a woman with four children why her figure was so stunning, she told me that she took an hour's exercise class three times a week; but that it was this particular exercise which she thought restored her flat stomach. So it's obviously worth persevering with, and it proves to me yet again that if you want a lovely figure, you must start exercising.

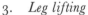

3. *Leg lifting*

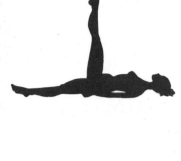

(a)   Also good for the tummy. Still lying on your back with your legs outstretched, lift and bend your right leg. Draw your knee up towards your chest, and straighten your leg pointing your toe towards the ceiling. Stretch it up as high as you can then slowly lower the straight leg to the ground. Repeat with the other leg.

This is a very easy but effective exercise. To make it more interesting, vary the rhythm and reverse the sequence. Do it in time to the music. Do not be over-zealous and try and lift both legs together. Although some people think this will do the job of strengthening the muscles faster, it doesn't – all it will do is to put a tremendous strain on the muscles of the lower back.

4. *Hip rolling*

(a)   Lie on your back with your knees up, feet on the floor. Roll your knees over from side to side touching the floor if you can. Try and keep your hips on the ground – and feel the muscles working in your waist.

5. *Bicycling in the air*

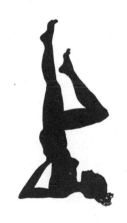

(a)   Supporting your hips, raise yourself up onto your shoulders and bicycle in the air – first one direction and then the other. Start slowly, then fast, then slowly again. This is another very well-known exercise which is great fun to do, and it's very good for the legs and hips.

If you aren't comfortable going up onto your shoulders, do the bicycling lying flat on your back with your legs above the ground. Whichever you choose, when bicycling remember to pedal your feet as well. To get the full benefit of this exercise, you must extend and flex the foot.

Some people may feel a strain in the lower back – if that is the case with you, stop immediately and do the following exercise instead.

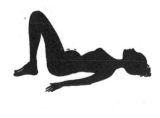

(b)   Lie flat on your back with your knees bent and your feet on the floor. Breathe in, fill yourself with air so that your stomach expands and pops up. Breathe out flattening your tummy and bringing your knees up to your chest. Repeat at least ten times. I was taught this exercise at an exercise class in Norway where they are very figure- and fitness-conscious. I was told that this exercise was far better than any bicycling and the very best way to flatten your stomach – and to learn how to breathe correctly.

I like both exercises. Try each of them and make your choice – or do them both.

6. *Side scissors*

(a)   Roll over onto your right side. Support your head on your out-stretched right arm, with your left hand on the ground in front of you.

Your hips should be well forward, and your body kept in a straight line throughout the exercise. Move your left leg and stretch it forward to touch the floor as far as you can. Then stretch the leg as far back as you can.

(b)   Now raise your left leg slowly up and down. If your hips are well forward, it is impossible to lift the leg right up, so just go as high as you can without straining. The idea is to stretch the muscles at the sides of the thighs and hips, not to do high kicks. Try first with the toe pointed, and then try with the foot flexed when you will feel the muscles pull more. Repeat ten times. Then roll over and repeat both exercises on the other side.

This exercise can be greatly improved by using weights strapped on-to your ankles. A beautiful Greek woman with firm slim thighs attributes them to leg lifting with weights. She is adamant that your foot should be flexed throughout the exercise. Exercise weights are available from good department stores, and are well worth getting, especially if your thighs need firming up.

7.   *Backward scissors*
(a)   Roll over onto your tummy. Rest your head on your hands. Stretch your right leg back and lift it up as high as you can while keeping your tummy and hips glued to the ground. Lower leg slowly and repeat with left leg. This is very good for hips, buttocks and backs of thighs. Repeat at least ten times.

8.   *The cobra*
(a)   Still on your tummy, with your hands tucked in under your shoulders and your forehead on the floor, raise your head until you can see the ceiling. Slowly raise your shoulders, pushing on your hands, raising your chest until your arms are straight, and your body is arched and stretched backwards. All the time keep staring at the ceiling, looking as far behind you as possible. Hold that curved position and then very slowly unroll yourself, stomach first, then chest, then shoulders, as though you are a carpet! Watch the ceiling until the very last minute. Relax in the starting position. Repeat three times. This is a marvellous exercise for the neck, back, and face, and the favourite of several enthusiastic exercisers whom I asked about it. So try it and see why.

'It is not enough to know,
One must also apply.
It is not enough to will to do
One must also do.'
Goethe

9. *Forward roll*

(a)   Roll over onto your back with your arms outstretched behind your head. Swing your body up and over into a sit-up, aim to touch your toes and try and touch your knees with your head. Then roll backwards, keeping your arms outstretched above your head, and bring your legs up and over to touch the floor behind you.

This is an easy relaxed roll, moving rhythmically backwards and forwards. If you are not very fit, do the exercise with bent knees, relax and enjoy it. As you get fitter you can aim to keep your knees straight and make it a more controlled exercise.

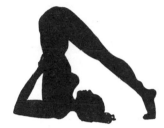

10.   *Shoulder stand*

(a)   This will relax you after that last energetic exercise. Lie on your back with your knees bent and feet on the ground. Lift your legs and body so that you are resting on your shoulders. Now try and lower your straight legs back until your feet are resting behind your head, and you form a triangle. You might find this difficult at first, so don't strain. Just go as far back as you can with comfort, and stay in that position. Then to relax your back and the backs of your legs, bend your knees down to the ground and try and clasp your head! This sounds odd but is amazingly relaxing.

Relaxers

Most people who are not very fit – which is most people! – should (very sensibly) take a few minutes to rest and relax after completing an exercise routine like the one I have just described. Instead of just lying gasping, why not try one of the relaxers that I describe below. There's no effort involved, just a constructive and practical use of the few minutes that all of us should allow for the body to come back to normal.

1.   *Deep breathing*

When asked to reveal her secret for a long life, the 80-year-old Sophie Tucker replied: 'Keep breathing.'

(a)   Lie flat on the floor with your head resting on a small pillow (or a couple of large books) and your knees bent and feet flat on the floor. Relax in that position, and concentrate on your breathing. Breathe out, and empty your lungs and stomach, flattening your stomach to help you. Breathe in, filling your lungs and diaphragm and expanding your tummy. In, out; in, out. Really fill your lungs full of air and then blow it out.

Do at least ten times. In fact, if you get tired during any of the exercising, do this deep breathing. Not only is it good for one's lungs but also one's tummy muscles. You can do this sitting, standing, or lying, so why not try and do it whenever you have an extra minute.

(b)   Lie on your side with your head on a pillow. Bend your knees up as close to your forehead as you can, clasping them with your arms to assist you. Hold that for a second and then relax in this curled up foetal position. Feel the spine stretching. This is a marvellous exercise – it's no effort, and is good for the back.

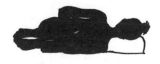

2. *Colours, floating*

Lie on the floor, relax, and let your breathing become gentle. Close your eyes and think of a colour. The first one that pops into your head. Imagine this colour enveloping you. Let it wash all over you. It sounds crazy, but try it, and see how marvellous it feels. Sometimes I imagine bright yellow and it's like being surrounded with lovely golden sun – very therapeutic on a cold winter day! Purple, or green or red; whatever colour you like. Do try it because it really is so lovely and relaxing.

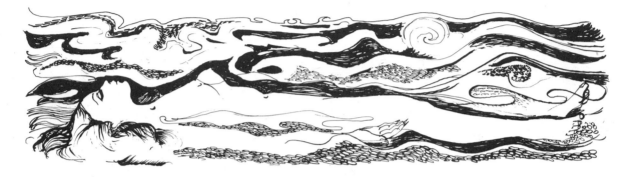

Belly-dancing

Now that you've mastered the exercises and do them every day – the warmers in the morning, the shapers in the evening (or whenever you have more time), and even know how to use your relaxing time constructively – you can try one of my favourite forms of exercise: belly-dancing.

The belly-dancing craze which swept the USA a few years ago has sound principles. It is not just a passing fad but an art form and an original and attractive way to exercise.

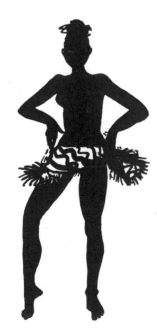

Belly-dancing can be done by anyone. You don't have to be a nymph to belly-dance. In fact, in the East, where belly-dancing originated, men and women of all ages, shapes and sizes do it. It is not dependent on any special figure type, although the women are frequently quite fat and voluptuous (which only goes to show that we are accustomed to too narrow a definition of beauty). Although there is no discrimination in age there is a slight discrimination in sex because men certainly don't make such good belly-dancers as women, but that hasn't stopped them trying!

First you need to find some music with a strong beat, preferably Oriental music, but African or reggae are also good. Any music with a definite rhythm and some drumming will do. You also need a scarf to tie tightly around your hips. This will help make you aware of the area you will be exercising and consequently make the dancing much easier.

Belly-dancing is both sexy and great fun. The most important things to remember when belly-dancing is that although your hips move freely, your head and shoulders and chest remain stationary. This is achieved by having slightly bent knees and rotating the hips. Imagine that your hips work independently of the rest of your body and have a life of their own.

Your hips ought to be *so* independent that you can balance something on your head while dancing. I recently saw a male dancer in a Greek restaurant who was enthusiastically gyrating to the music with a tray of six full wine-glasses balanced on his head!

Here are the basic movements which are much easier to do than they are to describe. It is really just a question of doing what comes naturally. Don't feel silly doing it. Practise by yourself in front of the mirror, and soon you will be ready to have people watching you with appreciation.

So put on the music, let go, and enjoy yourself.

1.   *The basic movement*

Stand with your feet about a foot apart. Your weight should be on your left leg, and your right leg should be bent slightly, the foot raised and balanced on the toes.

Push your right hip as far forward as possible and then circle to the left, side, behind and back to the front. Rotate the hips with a smooth undulating movement.

Practise this exaggerated circular action, then try changing the direction to see which way you find the easiest. Vary the speed and the size of the rotation to keep time to the music.

At first do this movement on the spot, and once you have mastered that try moving around the room, rotating and leading with your right foot and stepping with the left.

Once you can move across and around the room try making a turn. Keeping your left foot on the spot pivot around, still rotating your hips all the time.

2.   *Hip rotation*

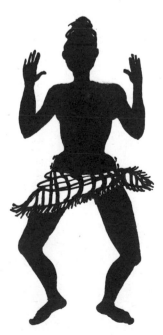

This is similar to the last movement but this time you are facing forward. Stand with your feet apart and your knees slightly bent. Swing your hips around in a large exaggerated circle. If you cannot get the rhythm of the complete circle break it up into smaller movements. First push your pelvis forward, then your hips out to the side, then as far back as possible and to the other side. Hit each point of the compass, north, east, south, west. Do several circles in one direction and then the other, all the time remembering to keep your upper body still and that only your hips are rotating. Keep the movement as fluid as possible – it's easy with a little practice.

3.   *The pelvic thrust*

Again standing with feet apart and knees slightly bent, contract the stomach and tilt the pelvis forward, which will pull your bottom up and under. Then roll your pelvis backwards pushing out your bottom and arching your back. This thrusting movement can be done either slowly or – how one usually sees it done, and the easiest way – very, very fast!

Many women I know have no flexibility in the pelvic area. This is because they are not using all their muscles. A belly-dancing friend told me that to get this thrusting movement and general flexibility one must contract the pelvic floor muscles (these are the muscles one uses when one is longing to go to the lavatory).

After having a baby the muscles become stretched and it is important to get these muscles into shape otherwise with age and lack of use one runs the risk of becoming incontinent. An added bonus of having these muscles in shape is that love-making becomes more enjoyable.

A marvellous gynaecologist told me this exercise to strengthen the pelvic floor muscles. Simply clench and relax all the muscles of the lower stomach and the vagina. You can do this isometric exercise anywhere and at any time. You can sit in the bus and at your desk and do it without anyone knowing. Just clench the muscles, hold the contraction and then let go. Do this ten times a day and you will definitely notice the difference. To get the pelvic thrust and general flexibility in the pelvic area *all* the muscles must be used in all the belly-dancing movements. It is the use of these pelvic muscles that makes the difference between just dancing and rotating the hips and actually *belly-dancing*.

In fact it is probably the use of these muscles, which are obviously so used in love-making, which makes belly-dancing so sexy.

4. *Belly rippling*

Some people can manage to make their bellies ripple. This rippling effect is obtained by contracting and relaxing the stomach muscles and is rather difficult to do. But it is a very good way of strengthening the stomach muscles and so worth a try.

5. *Shimmering and shaking*

This is simply a very fast, controlled shaking of the whole body so that you get a shimmering effect. Shake your shoulders and your bust as you sway from side to side from your hips. Although your whole body is shimmering and shaking your head is still held high and haughty! This sounds odd but can look very attractive. Keep in time with the music, and experiment.

With these basic movements you should easily be able to belly-dance. As I said, it really is only a matter of doing what comes naturally. Imagine that your hips have a life of their own, moving freely around your static body.

'Allah in his wisdom, made women perfect, except that he gave them tongues.'

Arabian proberb

Skin

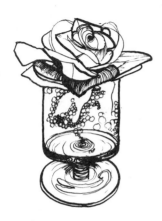

The skin is self-lubricating, self-cleaning and self-rejuvenating. If we were all to lead healthy lives in unpolluted and natural surroundings our skin would be able to look after itself quite adequately. But not many of us either live in a perfect environment, or have a perfect skin. We need to care for our skin, to balance its imperfections and counteract all the adverse conditions. Fortunately skin responds well to treatment, and consistent, conscientious care will give you good results. To achieve this improvement, however, we need to know a little about the skin and its functions.

The skin is not simply a waterproof wrapping, it is also a hardworking, highly efficient organ which weighs about six pounds and covers roughly seventeen feet. It eliminates waste in the form of sebum (the oil which lubricates our skin and hair), and water in the form of perspiration (this same process also regulates our temperatures). Thousands of tiny nerve endings provide us with a sense of touch. The skin breathes, and protects the body from the environment, the elements and bacteria.

There are two main layers, the dermis and the epidermis. The dermis is the lower layer, which is a jelly-like substance containing the oil and sweat glands, fat and blood cells, all supported by bundles of collagen fibres. With age these collagen fibres lose their flexibility and the skin loses some of its elasticity. (A tremendous amount of research is looking into ways in which to retard the skin's ageing process.) The dermis supports and nourishes the epidermis.

The epidermis is again divided into layers, the lower layer composed of plump, living cells, and the upper layer, the part we actually see, composed of flattened, horny, dead cells. The rounded living cells at the base divide and grow rapidly, pushing up towards the surface. These living, reproductive cells are nourished by the blood from the dermis and this is one of the many reasons why good circulation, exercise and diet are so essential if you want a good skin. As the cells move up, their protein content increases until the superficial dead layer (composed entirely of this protein, known as keratin) results. These flattened scale-like cells are constantly being shed and replaced by new ones – rather like the building of a wall. This continuous process of regeneration – every 20–30 days, depending on the individual – is known as mitosis.

As we grow older these upper dead cells do not shed so efficiently and so the skin can get a muddy look. We need to assist in the efficient removal of this dead skin as this will stimulate growth and improve the complexion. (See page 69 for ways in which to slough off dead skin cells.)

The surface cells require water to keep them moist and pliable, and this moisture is supplied by the dermis. Unfortunately this process – known as the Natural Moisturizing Factor – also becomes less efficient with age, and consequently the skin can become dehydrated, thereby needing more care.

Diet, exercise and sleep are all vitally important if you want a good skin.

Your diet should contain plenty of fresh fruit, vegetables and protein. Try to avoid eating too many carbohydrates, heavy sauces and highly spiced foods, as these can cause a pasty or spotty complexion. What you need is a plain, nutritionally well-balanced diet (our one on page 114 is ideal!).

Liquid is another very important ingredient in skin care. Drink as much as possible, at least eight glasses of water a day. This helps to clear the system and the result is a healthy, glowing skin.

Exercise and fresh air are also vitally important. As it is the blood that feeds the skin, if you increase your circulation by exercise there will obviously be an improvement in the skin itself. Ideally you should do some outdoor sport (to get the benefit of the fresh air), but if you live in a town, this can be difficult and so remember to do the warm-up exercises (page 147) every day, not only to improve your figure but also to make your skin glow with health.

I am a great advocate of the headstand, as this gets the blood rushing to the head. If a headstand is beyond you, try doing a shoulder stand or lying on a slant board (page 68).

Your emotions also greatly influence the state of your skin. If you are nervous, tired, depressed or in a bad temper, your hormones get so affected that the skin shows it by either coming up in a crop of spots, or looking pale and pasty. If you are feeling happy, calm and generally on top of the world, your skin also mirrors this, by looking alive and healthy. Maybe the answer is to be continually in love because that is often when the skin looks its most radiant!

The sebaceous glands are also mainly controlled by the hormones, which is why adolescents tend to have oily skins, and also explains why skin can become more oily during menstruation or at a time of emotional upheaval.

Too much fiddling around with your skin and constantly plastering your face with new cosmetics and make-up can have disastrous effects. I remember a beauty editor who came out in spots because she had been testing lots of different products, and it was all too much for her skin. Eventually she went to a dermatologist who told her to wash her face three times a day – nothing else. Now that her skin has cleared up she is still extremely careful. She washes her face and then applies diluted witch hazel, and occasionally she massages with the blandest of face creams. Her skin now looks beautiful because she has found the treatment that suits it best.

Sleep is another vital ingredient of good skin. It's *not* a myth that 'you need your beauty sleep'. It is *essential*. You only have to look at your skin after a night without sleep to verify this (page 132).

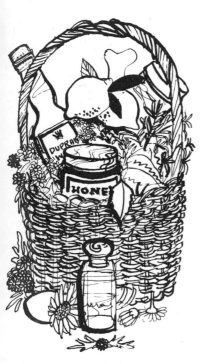

'A woman who could always be in love would never grow old.'
Richter

Your skin type

A tremendous amount is written about the different types of skin and all the different products they need. I feel a lot of this is unnecessary, as it is really just a question of common sense. If your skin feels greasy, wash it frequently; and if it feels dry, lubricate it.

As I have said, your skin is always changing – due to the weather, your age, or your emotional state. Sometimes it will feel dry, another time greasy, and you must learn to vary your skin care to suit your needs. You must be aware of the condition of your skin so that you can change your routine to suit it.

To discover your type simply study your face carefully in a mirror.

Dry skin

This is usually pretty, fine and delicately textured. It can feel as though it is pulled too tightly over your bones. It can also have a tendency to broken veins, dry patches and tiny lines which if neglected turn into wrinkles, and so it needs lots of pampering and lubricating. This type also tends to be sensitive and allergic and so it should be treated with mild preparations. Check your diet – do you eat enough fat and protein? Try to eat some oily fish (sardines) or take cod liver oil tablets which really help improve dry skin.

Greasy skin

This tends to look slightly sallow and shiny. The grease picks up dirt and clogs the pores. Blackheads form, which, if neglected, can turn into spots and blemishes. In the long run this is a good skin, because with age, skin becomes drier, and being thicker, greasy skin doesn't line as easily and it retains its elasticity.

However, it needs frequent, meticulous cleaning. Watch your diet and try and avoid oily, spicy or rich food. Doctors now say that chocolate is off the list of forbidden food but people who suffer from greasy skin tell me they find a correlation, and so I'd advise you to stay away from it – better for your figure too!

Combination skin

This is the most common skin type – dry cheeks, neck and eye area, and a greasy patch down the centre. You must try to balance the two types of complexion, by adding cream and moisture to the dry area and removing excess grease, with extra washing, from the oily panel. Treat your skin for the prevalent condition and just pay a little extra attention to the other parts.

Basic skin care

Everyone knows that they must cleanse, tone and cream – but I am going to tell you why.

There are no hard and fast rules for skin care. The vital thing is to find out what suits *your* skin. But having said that, I do think that if you want a good skin, you must keep it clean. There are two different

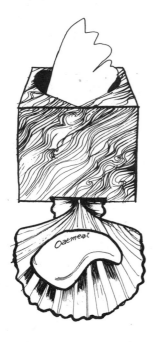

ways of cleaning the skin – washing it, and cleansing it with cream. Both are necessary.

Washing

Contrary to many present-day popular beliefs, the older I get the more I believe in washing the face.

When I trained as a beauty therapist, we were taught never to wash our faces – soap and water were most definitely out. But in the last few years, after working with many different skin types, I now believe it to be beneficial to the skin – even dry skin. Washing your face is the simplest beauty treatment you can give yourself. If your skin is very fine and sensitive wash with water alone. When washing with soap, massage the lather into the skin, working with your finger tips in upward circular movements. I am against face cloths as they can all too easily get dirty. Make sure you rinse your face thoroughly – at least five times with warm water – until all traces of soap have gone. Blot your face dry with a tissue. In this way you again ensure complete hygiene.

How frequently you should wash your face will depend entirely on how you feel. Sometimes you might find that you want to wash it three times a day, whereas another week, if your skin feels slightly dry, it may be only once. As a general guide I think all of us ought to wash our face first thing in the morning. But as with all skin care, each skin is individual. Only *you* can decide what suits you.

So once again, the only absolute hard and fast rule is that if you want a good skin you must keep it clean.

Orange and oatmeal washing grains

2 tablespoons oatmeal
1 tablespoon ground orange peel

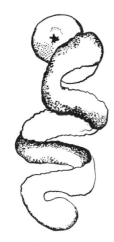

Some people find that washing with soap is too harsh for their skin so washing with grains is an excellent alternative. Of all the cosmetics I make, I think that these grains are the most popular. They suit all skin types. The oatmeal cleanses the face marvellously, imparting a lovely sheen to the skin. A Kashmiri friend told me about this use of orange peel and I will be forever grateful to her, as it not only smells heavenly but has a slightly toning and abrasive action on the skin. Dry the orange peels in the sun, or in a very, very slow oven, or on top of a storage heater and then grind them up in a coffee grinder.

Mix the ground orange peel with the oatmeal and put into a pretty wide necked bottle (an old herb jar is ideal). To use, pour about a handful into the palm of your hand, moisten this into a paste and use it to wash with. The scrubbing effect of the grains leaves your skin looking and feeling wonderfully clean, and sparkling with health.

If you feel lazy and can't be bothered to dry and grind the orange peel simply use the oatmeal – it's still good but doesn't smell nearly as exotic.

Cornmeal, sunflower and almond meal are also all very good to wash with.

Facial scrubs

Apart from washing with grains, you can also give yourself a facial scrub.

One easy way is to add a teaspoon of your washing grains to a teaspoon of double cream or honey. Massage this paste really well into the skin. In this mixture the grains are more abrasive than when you simply mix them with water, and this means that you can really work the granules into the skin. This thoroughly cleanses the skin, dislodges any dirt, sloughs off dead skin and will improve a sluggish complexion. You will be amazed at the amount of dirt that comes rolling off – an easy way of giving yourself a mini face peeling. It leaves the skin glowing with health and satiny smooth.

Cleansing with creams

To remove make-up you need to cleanse with a cleansing cream or milk. It is no use trying to remove make-up by washing, as it is waterproof, and no amount of washing will be able to remove it properly.

Apply your cream or lotion lavishly, massage it in, and then remove with dampened cotton wool. Don't use tissues as they are not really as absorbent as cotton wool and being paper (originally made from wood), they can scratch the skin.

All the following recipes have been tried and tested and we have found them to be quick and easy to make. Making your own cosmetics has many advantages, one of them being that, after the initial outlay for ingredients, it is infinitely cheaper. It also means that you can use the very best of everything; the best oils, for instance – wheatgerm, almond and avocado – which, because of their cost, and the fact that they can go rancid, a commercial firm would be unable to use in anything like the same quantity.

If you follow these recipes carefully you will find that you will be able to make creams that are as good as (or better than) any you could buy.

In these recipes I have included a few drops of essential oil to make the cosmetics smell as good as they look, but this addition is entirely optional. Commercial products are often heavily perfumed and it can be this which contributes to skin allergies. By using essential oils to scent the creams an allergic reaction is unlikely, but if your skin is very sensitive just leave it out.

Preservatives are not included in these recipes and so they only have a shelf life of about three months. This can be extended if you keep the creams in the refrigerator and so if you make a large quantity keep the bulk in the refrigerator and a small jar out ready for use. But the whole idea of home-made cosmetics is to use them while they are still fresh – so use them really lavishly and enjoy yourself.

It is also extremely important to put labels on the jar of finished cream – I always think I will remember what it is, but never do! In fact if you want to be really efficient keep a notebook (or write in the margin here beside the recipe) of how it turned out and your comments. So, always label your pots and bottles *immediately* after you put the lid on them.

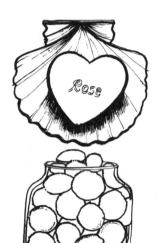

'Cleanliness is half a virtue and uncleanliness is a vice and a half.'
Dumas

1 tablespoon white
   beeswax
1 tablespoon petroleum
   jelly (Vaseline)
10 teaspoons mineral oil
   (3 tablespoons + 1
   teaspoon)

2 tablespoons boiled (or
   bottled) water
¼ teaspoon borax
2 drops verbena oil

Verbena cleansing cream

Melt the wax, vaseline and mineral oil together over a water bath and in a separate bowl, dissolve the borax in the boiled water. When the wax has melted, slowly add the water and borax to the oils. Remove the bowl from the heat and stir it until it sets. I always use an electric beater (on low speed) because it makes the process quicker, but it is quite possible to stir. When it is nearly cool add in the verbena oil which makes it smell marvellously fresh. Incidentally, in medieval times verbena was used for warding off the powers of witches and enchanters.

This makes about a cup of firm, snowy white cream which liquifies on touching the skin. Use it generously for removing make-up.

1½ tablespoons beeswax
1 tablespoon emulsifying
   wax
4 tablespoons mineral oil

5 tablespoons boiled (or
   bottled) water
¼ teaspoon borax
1 tablespoon witch hazel

1 drop lavender oil

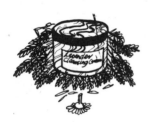

Lavender cleansing cream

Melt the waxes and oil together over a water bath. At the same time in a separate bowl, dissolve the borax in the boiled water and then add the witch hazel. Remove both bowls from the heat and mix the waters into the oils, stirring continuously, or beat until it starts to thicken. When the cream is beginning to cool add in a drop of lavender so that it smells refreshing each time you use it. The word lavender comes from the Latin *lavare* – to wash – and so its use seems most suited to a cleansing cream.

We use mineral oil because it doesn't penetrate the skin, which makes it perfect for removing make-up and dirt, and the witch hazel because it gives the cream a slightly astringent quality.

This is one of my favourite cleansing creams, and is as good as any commercial cream. These quantities make about a cup of soft airy cream.

1 tablespoon beeswax
2 tablespoons coconut oil
4 tablespoons mineral oil
1 teaspoon stearic acid
   (optional)

2 tablespoons boiled water
   or lemon juice
1 tablespoon witch hazel
¼ teaspoon borax

2 drops lemon oil

Lemon and coconut cleansing cream

Melt waxes and oils over a water bath and slowly add in the heated water and witch hazel in which you have dissolved the borax. Stir continuously until it cools, then add in the lemon oil and continue stirring until it begins to set.

This makes a rather greasy, slightly old-fashioned cream. With the addition of the stearic acid to the waxes and then 2 extra tablespoons of water you will bet a much more modern cream – very light, fluffy and easy to use.

I have given you both versions because some of you may have difficulty in obtaining stearic acid – but do try and persuade your chemist to get it for you, as I have included it in several recipes. Stearic acid is a natural fatty acid which gives a pearliness to creams.

Toning

A skin tonic makes your skin feel marvellously refreshed and clean. You can use either a tonic, which is usually a mild aromatic water, or an astringent which tends to be stronger and often contains alcohol. Personally I am not in favour of very strong astringents – the use of a lot of alcohol is too harsh and will dry out even a greasy skin. I think that it is much better to use a milder tonic liberally than a strong astringent.

One good reason for using a skin tonic is to help to restore the skin's acid mantle. Our skin has a thin film of acid matter covering it, which acts as a barrier and protects the skin from infection. The acidity is measured on a pH scale which runs from 0–14: numbers 0–7 represent acidity and 7–14 alkalinity. The pH of the skin ranges from 3–5·5 and so ideally we should apply tonics of about this acidity. If the level of acidity or alkalinity of the skin is too high it can make the skin itch – one simple remedy for this is to add a teaspoon of vinegar to the bath.

In a normal healthy skin the acid balance rapidly restores itself. For instance it will return to its natural acid state within 2–4 hours after washing with soap and water. But we can help this process, first by making sure that after washing, the skin is completely free from all traces of soap – you must rinse thoroughly. And also after using a cleansing cream remove all traces of that with a skin tonic.

Skin tonics are the easiest of cosmetics to make and all the following recipes require no exotic ingredients. You probably already have everything needed in the kitchen.

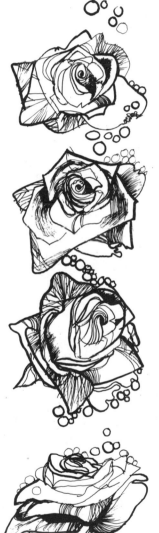

Rose water

Rose water is acclaimed all over the world as the queen of the flower waters. You can buy rose water from any chemist and if your skin is dry use it by itself, or if your skin is greasy mix it with witch hazel – $\frac{2}{3}$ rose water to $\frac{1}{3}$ witch hazel. This is not only the easiest and most renowned of skin tonics, but also one of the very best.

Roses have been used for healing for centuries. It is said that Milto, a fair young maiden, daughter of an artisan, deposited fresh garlands of roses in the temple of Venus. Her beauty became threatened by a tumour on her chin, but she saw in a dream the goddess telling her to apply to it some of the roses from the altar. She did so, and recovered her charms so completely that she eventually sat on the Persian throne as the favourite wife of Cyrus. Since then, roses have formed the basis of many lotions.

Witch hazel

This is also an invaluable ingredient in skin tonics, because of its astringent properties. In Brazil it is known as 'miraculous cure-all', and is used as an antiseptic, and to reduce swellings and puffiness. A friend in France tells me it is still also greatly used in Europe. One day she caught her hand in the car door and was in absolute agony until she remembered witch hazel. Almost miraculously, the pain and swelling disappeared. And the beauty editor of one of the best-known magazines tells me that she uses practically nothing but witch hazel – it's virtually her only cosmetic.

Vinegar

Another useful ingredient in skin tonics. Dilute one part vinegar to eight parts water. This acidic water can be used as a skin tonic, in the bath or as a final rinse when washing your hair.

The smell of plain vinegar leaves something to be desired and you can easily make it more aromatic by adding herbs and dried flowers.

To a cup of cider or wine vinegar add 2 tablespoons lavender, 1 tablespoon tarragon, ½ teaspoon cloves, 1 tablespoon rose petals – in fact any herb or flowers you like the smell of. Leave to stand for two weeks, shaking the bottle daily, then strain the vinegar, dilute it and use it lavishly. It will be a beautiful colour with a wonderful perfume.

1 tablespoon each of absinthe leaves, rosemary leaves, sage leaves, mint leaves, cinnamon, grated nutmeg
½ cup vodka
1 cup white wine vinegar

A Belgian friend found this spicy vinegar recipe in her grandmother's handwritten book of recipes. We tried it diluted (8 parts water to 1 part vinegar) as a skin tonic and can thoroughly recommend it. Cut or crush the herb leaves and put them into a large wide topped bottle or jar, add the spices and alcohol. Tightly close the bottle and leave it in the sun for two weeks. Then filter and add the vinegar. Shake well, then re-filter.

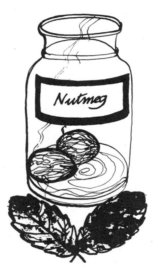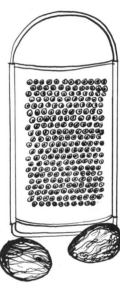

Rosemary tonic

In 1555 Master Alexis the Piedmontese recorded the following recipe. 'To Make the Face Fair, Take the fresh blossoms of rosemary and boil them in white wine; then wash the face with it and use it as a drink – and you shall make your face very fair and your breath sweet.'

Rosemary has a stimulating effect on the skin and according to some stories it was through the use of a rosemary skin tonic that Queen Elizabeth of Hungary retained her beauty, and at the age of seventy-two her hand was asked for in marriage.

1 cup white wine
4 tablespoons dried rosemary
1 drop orange oil
2 drops lemon oil

I have adapted the old recipes to make this one. Mix all these together, let them stand for about a week, shaking frequently. Strain and bottle. It smells lovely, but if you find it too strong dilute with a little orange-flower water.

Culpeper has this to say about rosemary and so I use it frequently in the hope that it really will work – 'It helps weak memory and quickens the senses. It is very comfortable to the stomach in all cold maladies.'

Cucumber tonic

½ cucumber
2 tablespoons witch hazel
1 tablespoon alcohol
   (optional)

Cucumbers have the same pH as the skin and so their use as a skin freshener is most beneficial. Cut the cucumber up into chunks and liquidize it. Strain, and then add the witch hazel. This makes a lovely refreshing skin tonic. The only drawback is that cucumbers go bad rather quickly. The witch hazel makes it last slightly longer, but you should keep it in the refrigerator and use it up quickly. If your skin is greasy you could add a tablespoon of alcohol which would also extend the life of the cucumber but it is still wise to store it in the refrigerator. I sometimes add a couple of drops of peppermint extract (or mint leaves) to this tonic to make it even more refreshing and tingly.

½ cucumber
6 tablespoons orange-
   flower water
1½ tablespoons alcohol
3 tablespoons purified
   water

The advantage of this next cucumber tonic is that it will keep for a couple of weeks. It is extremely refreshing and leaves the skin feeling soft and cool. Peel and cut the cucumber into slices, and cook them slowly in a double boiler. When soft, sieve the cucumber to squeeze out all the juice. Mix this juice with the alcohol and orange-flower water. Shake them all together and the tonic is ready.

Incidentally, if you are ever going on a long journey, I would recommend you take a few cucumbers. Last year when I was travelling around Afghanistan by bus, they proved immensely useful. On our long journeys, we became extremely hot and dusty. We peeled the cucumbers, and the vegetable quenched our thirst and satisfied our hunger while the inside of the peel was perfect for cleaning our hot faces and wiping our sticky hands.

So remember, cucumbers make the perfect beauty treatment, both cooling and refreshing. (And incidentally, as if all these qualities were not enough, I also read that cucumbers contain a hormone which is an anti-wrinkle aid!)

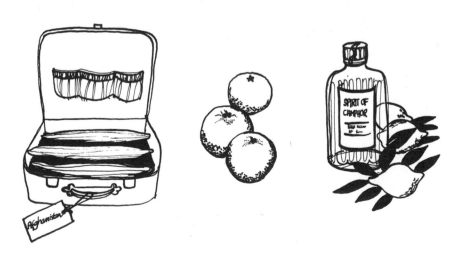

Orange and lemon tonic

½ cup orange-flower water
½ cup witch hazel
¼ cup lemon juice
1 cup purified (or bottled) water
1 tablespoon alcohol (vodka)
2 drops camphor spirit
2 drops lemon or orange oil

Mix all the ingredients together in a large bottle and shake vigorously. All the witch hazel, orange and lemon juice make this a marvellously refreshing skin tonic, and it takes only a couple of minutes to make. The camphor, which smells terrific, is a soothing and anti-inflammatory agent, especially good for spotty skin and open pores.

This tonic is suitable for normal and greasy skin, but the lemon juice and alcohol make it slightly too strong for very dry skin.

Tingly astringent or after-shave lotion

1½ tablespoons witch hazel
1 tablespoon alcohol (vodka)
½ tablespoon glycerine
⅛ teaspoon alum
small pinch of menthol crystals
¾ cup boiled water
drop of blue colouring
1–2 drops essential oil

Dissolve the alum and menthol crystals in the boiled water, then add the glycerine, witch hazel and vodka. Add a drop of blue colouring and a couple of drops of your favourite essential oil – last time I made it I used jasmine.

I add alum to this recipe for its astringent qualities, and in fact you can add it to any of the preceding recipes if you would like them to be stronger.

This astringent really brings the blood to the surface and leaves the skin literally tingling. It is ideal for greasy skin or for an after-shave.

Moisturizing and nourishing creams

Both these terms are actually misnomers, as their action is still open to debate. If we were to be pedantic about it, we would call them lubricating creams.

Some doctors and chemists say that the main purpose of a cream, whether a moisturizer or a rich night cream, is to prevent moisture loss. They maintain that the oils and moisture are not absorbed by the skin and that the creams we apply simply prevent moisture loss by holding the natural moisture in our skin. Whereas, quite obviously, the cosmetic manufacturers tell us that the creams are absorbed and are replacing water loss and pumping up our tissues.

Frankly, I don't think it really matters which is correct – there is probably truth in both theories. All we need to know is that we must apply cream to keep our skins looking smooth, soft, moist and supple.

For this reason I am putting all the creams together – I really do not believe in a day or a night cream. I think it depends on what your skin wants. If your skin feels very dry, put on a richer cream, and if it feels normal, a lighter one – it is purely a question of preference.

We have all been brainwashed into wanting specific creams for specific reasons but if you know anything about the skin this is nonsense – it depends entirely on what your skin needs at the time. You eat what you like, when you like, so I think you should treat your skin in the same way.

Light rose cream

Melt the wax, lanolin and almond oil together in an enamel or Pyrex bowl over a water bath. In a separate bowl heat the rose water, borax

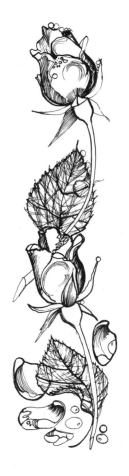

2 tablespoons emulsifying
   wax
1 teaspoon lanolin
2 tablespoons almond oil

8 tablespoons rose water
3 tablespoons witch hazel
½ teaspoon glycerine
¼ teaspoon borax

2 drops rose oil

and glycerine and when the borax is dissolved add in the witch hazel. Remove the bowls from the heat and slowly add the waters to the oils. Beat on the low speed of your electric beater, or stir continuously until the cream begins to cool and thicken, then add in the rose oil.

These quantities give you about a cup of soft, white cream. It is a very light non-greasy cream, ideal for all skin types (and even for men), which can be used by itself or under make-up. Roses are said to have aphrodisiac properties which could make the daily use of this cream even more beneficial!

> *The Rose distils a healing balm*
> *The beating pulse of pain to calm.*
> Anacreon, 6th century BC

Avocado and orange cream

1 tablespoon beeswax (or
   paraffin wax)
½ teaspoon stearic acid
2 tablespoons avocado oil
2 tablespoons sunflower
   oil

2 tablespoons orange-
   flower (or boiled) water
⅛ teaspoon borax

2 drops orange-flower oil

Melt the oils and waters separately over a water bath. Remove from the heat and slowly add the water (making sure that the borax has been completely dissolved, otherwise your cream may feel gritty). Beat or stir the cream until it starts to cool, and then add a couple of drops of orange-flower oil. Continue stirring until you get a firm, glossy cream.

This makes about one cup of delicious cream which is absorbed into the skin almost instantly.

Orange-flower water and oil make the cream smell heavenly. The custom of using orange blossoms for brides dates to the time of the Saracen ladies who wore blossoms on their wedding day in the hope that they would be as fruitful as the orange tree! (The Crusaders brought back this custom of using orange flowers to Europe and it has gradually spread world wide.)

Rich wheatgerm cream

1 tablespoon lanolin
   (anhydrous)
1 tablespoon beeswax
1 tablespoon emulsifying
   wax
4 tablespoons wheatgerm
   oil
2 tablespoons almond oil

8 tablespoons boiled (or
   bottled) water
⅛ teaspoon borax (optional)

2 drops tincture of benzoin
2 drops orange or lemon
   oil

Melt the waxes and heat the waters in the usual way. Remove the bowls from the heat and slowly, stirring all the time, add the waters to the waxes and oils. When the cream cools, add in the tincture of benzoin and orange oil and continue beating until it sets.

This makes about a cup of fine, rich cream. We use lanolin (wool fat) because it is a terrific emollient. However, a few people are allergic to lanolin and so if you find that this cream does not suit you, that is probably the reason. The other problem with lanolin is that it is very sticky to handle and has a rather persistent smell. But I think that its skin softening and moisturizing qualities outweigh all these slight inconveniences.

In this cream we have used a large quantity of wheatgerm oil (vitamin E) which has a tremendously nourishing effect on the skin. Wheatgerm also has a rather nutty smell which people either love or hate – so in this recipe I've used lemon or orange oil, both fairly strong, to mask both the smell of the lanolin and the wheatgerm. But don't let my pointing out these problems deter you from making this marvellous cream. It really is one of the best, richest creams you could possibly make, ideal if your skin feels neglected or dry.

Rich lecithin and sandalwood cream

2 teaspoons beeswax
½ teaspoon stearic acid
½ teaspoon lanolin
¼ teaspoon lecithin oil (optional)
2 tablespoons sesame (or safflower) oil

3 tablespoons water (boiled or bottled)
⅛ teaspoon borax

2–4 drops of sandalwood oil

Melt the waxes and oils in a bowl over a water bath and dissolve the borax in the heated water in a separate bowl. Remove the bowls from the heat and slowly, stirring all the time, add the water to the oils. When it is cool add in the sandalwood oil and continue stirring until it sets. This gives you about three-quarters of a cup of lovely pale cream which is extremely nourishing. It seems to cling to the skin giving it a lovely sheen.

In this recipe we have rich oil and lecithin. I added the lecithin as it is a natural emulsifier and helps smooth the skin. It is best to use lecithin oil (which should be available from a good health shop, or you can squeeze it out of a lecithin capsule), but if it's simply not available you could use lecithin granules (the ones that I hope you are eating with your breakfast cereal, page 63). Mix ¼ teaspoon lecithin granules with ¼ teaspoon boiling water and add this dissolved lecithin to the cream before it cools. You can greatly increase the effectiveness of any creams by adding a dash of lecithin to them.

I have used sandalwood in the cream for two reasons – one, because it smells wonderful and will mask the rather heavy smell of the lanolin, and two, because it is a beauty treatment in itself. In India I was told that if I wanted to have smooth, soft, wrinkle-free skin I should apply sandalwood oil each night. The recipe I was given is to mix four drops of pure sandalwood oil (Mysore is the best) with a tablespoon of olive oil and a few drops of lemon juice. I tried this recipe and it smelt so exotic and luxuriant that I felt sure it must be beneficial. Another use of sandalwood was given to me by an Indian doctor who said that sandalwood paste was one of the very best cures for spots, rashes and even newly formed scars. You make this paste by rubbing a stick of sandalwood in some milk on a marble slab. The ensuing paste is used on any skin blemishes. A friend from Ceylon also swears by this same paste.

Masks

Masks are marvellous things. They are so easy to make and there are so many different ones just waiting in the kitchen for you to mix up and use.

Masks are the perfect pick-me-up to both your spirits and your skin – they make you feel pampered. They can be used every day, once a week, or whenever you feel like a treat. Apply the mixture to the face and leave it on for about ten or twenty minutes. The ideal is to relax whilst the mask is on – lie down and put your feet up. But I know this isn't always possible, so don't *not* put on a mask just because you have no time to relax. You could have it on while having your bath or doing the cooking.

Masks date back to the Pharaohs of Egypt and were part of the cult of Isis. The first accurate details of any recipes are those of the fourth century recorded by Ovid. His formulae tell us how to mix wool wax (our lanolin) with honey, eggs, powdered narcissi bulbs, orris powder and excrement of sea birds into a mask to 'obtain a sparkling face' and do away with freckles.

Poppaea, Nero's wife, revealed her own personal formula only a few days before she died. She kept her mixture – the basis of which was milk – on her face for several days. It was considered to greatly improve the complexion and was named Poppaenum after her.

Here is a selection of my favourite masks, but remember that these are only basic examples. I hope that you will soon be experimenting to find out what really suits your own skin.

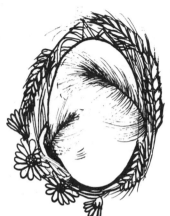

Egg masks

'In marble walls as white as milk
Lined with skin as soft as silk
Within a fountain crystal clear
A golden apple doth appear
No doors there are to this stronghold
Yet thieves break in and steal the gold
What is it?
An egg.'

The egg is one of the most famous and the best of face masks. The whole egg can be used: the yolk contains lecithin and protein and is nourishing; the egg white is slightly drying and astringent.

If your skin is normal use the whole egg, with 1 teaspoon honey and 1 teaspoon almond oil. If your skin is dry use only the egg yolk, mixing it with honey and wheatgerm oil. If your skin is greasy use only the egg white. Whisk it up with a couple of drops of almond oil and apply. Although the egg white is slightly drying it is an ideal as a 'pre-party tightener' – it reduces any puffiness, and only temporarily (I'm afraid) reduces wrinkles.

Whisk the egg in all these recipes because the air in the egg makes it nicer to apply.

Incidentally, eggs are not only useful as face masks, they also make a terrific 'beauty' food. They are an excellent source of protein, containing all the essential amino acids. They contain copper, iron, phosphorous and vitamins A, B, D and E. Raw eggs, however, should not be eaten in great quantity because the white contains a substance (ovidin) which if taken excessively can be harmful. (This ovidin is destroyed by heat.)

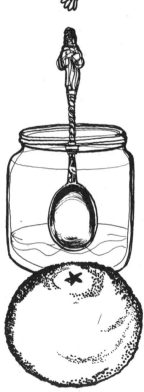

1 tablespoon yoghurt
1 tablespoon brewers' yeast
1 teaspoon oatmeal
1 teaspoon honey
1 teaspoon orange juice or cider vinegar

Yoghurt masks

Plain yoghurt can be used, just as it is, as a cleansing face mask – in Turkey I was told that anyone with acne should use this mask every day and that it would soon clear the skin of blemishes. Many clients and their children have since proved that this is true.

Yoghurt is also useful as a base for other ingredients. Try mixing it with honey and oatmeal and brewers' yeast or soft fruit – in fact anything you happen to have in the kitchen and you like the sound of.

Mix all these ingredients together and apply the thick paste to your face. Let it dry and then wash it off with warm water. The brewers' yeast has a stimulating effect on the skin. It can, however, bring impurities to the surface, and so don't use this mask just before a party until you know how it reacts on your skin. This is a terrific mask, leaving the skin feeling firm, smooth and clean.

As you can see you may apply almost the same things to your face as you eat. This mask is almost identical to your breakfast cereal – in fact you could easily use that as a face mask. Just mix it into a paste with a little milk, cream or yoghurt!

Milk mask

2 tablespoons dried milk
1 tablespoon rose water
½ tablespoon wheatgerm oil

Mix all the ingredients together into a paste. If you like a smooth paste first dissolve the dried milk in the rose water or if you like a slight grittiness, mix with the wheatgerm oil first. Leave it on your face fifteen minutes and then rub it off by damping your fingertips and then rubbing them in circles all over the face.

Do this over a basin because it makes a terrible mess, but it is worth the mess as it sloughs off dead skin and lots of dirt. This mask leaves your skin smooth, shiny, soft and glowing with health.

Honey

Honey is an invaluable aid to health and beauty. It is a natural moisturizer, healer, soother and skin softener. In face masks, it can be used just as it is, but is rather too sticky, so it is better combined with various other ingredients. It makes a marvellous binder, and can be used in absolutely any recipe you come across (as you can see I have already used it in the preceding two recipes). Honey can also be added to any of the face or body creams that you make. Only add a little at first, as it can make them feel a little tacky, which some people don't like.

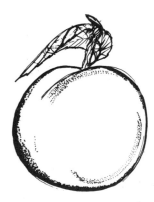

½ peach
1 teaspoon double cream
½ teaspoon honey

Peach mask

In ancient China peaches were originally called 'fairy fruit'. They were the symbol of immortality because, according to legend, the peach tree grew in the mythical gardens, and the fruit was the sacred food of the eight Taoist Immortals.

Hoping for an 'immortal skin' I thought I'd include this face mask. Finely mash the peach and mix it with the cream and honey. This is a nourishing mask which smells absolutely wonderful, leaving your skin with the proverbial 'peaches and cream' complexion.

1 tablespoon kaolin (or Fuller's earth)
1 tablespoon milk or rose water
1 teaspoon olive oil
A couple of drops of lemon juice

Mud packs

Mud was used by ancient civilizations to beautify the skin. In some areas this practise still continues and you hear of the 'special' mud or clay from a particular area. The property of these muds is that they cleanse the skin, or hair, thoroughly, without stripping off its natural oils.

These special earths are full of minerals, and in Fez, where it is called *ghrassoul*, a woman gave me some which she always mixed with rose and jasmine petals. But we don't need to be so exotic. All we need to do is to go to the chemist and buy either kaolin or Fuller's earth. Mix all the ingredients into a paste and apply it. These mud packs clean and refine the skin, giving it a lovely glow and fine texture.

Strawberry mask

4 strawberries
1 tablespoon double
  cream

Strawberries are another fruit which make a marvellous face mask. They are acidic, and have a slightly bleaching effect on the skin. Mash the strawberries, strain them through a sieve, and mix the juice with the double cream. There's no excuse, during the strawberry season, not to use this simple mask frequently. Every time you buy strawberries to eat, keep a few aside and make up this delicious mask – you can always eat any of the mixture that's left!

Lecithin mask

Lecithin is very useful, because of its nourishing ability. Dissolve a teaspoon of lecithin granules in a teaspoon of orange juice if your skin is slightly greasy, or a teaspoon of milk if your skin is dry. Or add it to the following fruit masks.

Avocado mask

1 tablespoon avocado
1 teaspoon honey
2 drops lemon juice

A really nourishing, easy and luxuriant mask can be made by simply mashing up some avocado pear. Mash and sieve the avocado and then add in the honey and lemon juice. If you think it is a waste to use avocado on the skin, buy those very mushy ones from the greengrocers and use them – it doesn't matter how black they are.

This mask is especially good for dry skin. Bananas can be used in the same way, as they contain vitamin A and also make a marvellous, nourishing face mask.

Mayonnaise

1 egg yolk
1 tablespoon cider vinegar
½ cup sunflower oil

Home-made mayonnaise (or even bought mayonnaise as long as it does not contain preservatives) makes a marvellous face mask. It contains all the ingredients for a really good mask: egg for nourishing, oil for lubricating and the vinegar for its acidic value. Mix the egg yolk and vinegar together first and then slowly add in the oil. I usually add a tablespoon of honey just to make it even more beneficial to the skin. This makes enough mayonnaise for several masks – put the remainder into a *labelled* jar and store it in the refrigerator. It can also be the base for a fruit mask. Just mash up the fruit and add it to a tablespoon of mayonnaise. Tomatoes, strawberries, apples, cucumbers, avocado and herbs can all be added.

Paw-paw mask

In 1977 the value of the paw-paw (papaya) was dramatically demonstrated. A kidney transplant patient, at a London hospital, had developed a post-operative infection which was cured by the paw-paw. Its application healed the infected wound when antibiotics had failed. Strips of the fruit were laid over the wound and it healed rapidly. The doctor in charge had been in South Africa and seen Africans applying paw-paw to ulcers and wounds. Since then he had used it successfully on several patients.

In Kenya I always use a mask of paw-paw. After my daily breakfast of half a paw-paw, I rub the inside skin all over my face, and I can see an improvement in my complexion after a few days.

Carrot mask

1 medium-sized carrot
1 tablespoon honey

Boil the sliced carrot in a very little water. When it is soft enough mash it up and mix it with the honey and apply.

This slightly crazy mask is very effective and well worth trying especially if you happen to have any blemishes. Carrots are strongly antiseptic and in country remedies, were sometimes used as poultices on ulcers.

So we should not only eat carrots, for all their vitamin A, we should also apply them to our faces. Recently I came across yet another use for them. The ladies of fashion, during the reign of James I used its feathery leaves in their head-dresses! Obviously carrots have endless possibilities!

I have given you some suggestions and recipes for various masks but obviously you can easily make up your own recipes. Here is a list of the various ingredients that are most commonly used, so that you can experiment for yourself. Have fun.

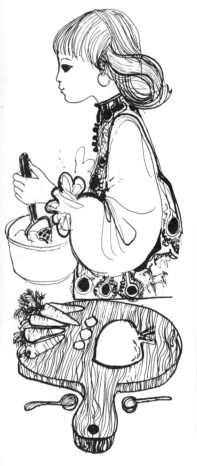

Thickeners and binders	Bases	Fruit and vegetable
powdered milk	yoghurt	apple
oatmeal	milk	banana
kaolin	cream	avocado
lecithin	mayonnaise	carrot
Fuller's earth		peach
orange peel		strawberries
brewers yeast		herbs
honey		onion
eggs		tomato
		paw-paw

Are you making the most of yourself?

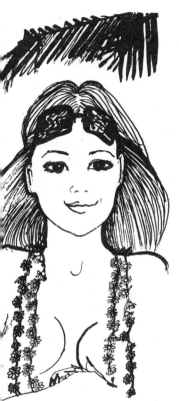

By now you should be feeling, and looking marvellous. You will have studied your face and your figure in the Mirror Tests and you should know all your good and bad points. It is now time to examine your image – are you making the most of yourself?

MAXIMIZE YOUR GOOD POINTS AND MINIMIZE THE BAD

Make a mental note of the type of clothes you are wearing when you get the most compliments and design your wardrobe around those styles. Don't copy anyone else. What suits them will not necessarily suit you. A friend, a well-known dress designer, is always bemoaning the fact that people slavishly follow fashion instead of adapting it to suit themselves. Her hint on how to look beautiful is only to have clothes in your wardrobe that actually flatter you. She's always telling me that it is better to have a *few flattering clothes* than *masses* of ill-assorted bits and pieces. In other words, you should throw out anything that does not flatter you.

KNOW THE COLOURS THAT SUIT YOU BEST

Find out which colours emphasize your eyes and flatter your skin and hair. Make these 'flatterers' the basic colours of your wardrobe. You obviously don't want to wear only one colour but it is very useful to know what suits you, and it is lovely getting compliments. (Incidentally reds, oranges and yellows tend to increase your size and blues and greens and mauves decrease it.)

DEVELOP YOUR OWN IMAGE

If you like something whether it is fashionable or not, wear it. Make your own style. For instance, some men have enormous collections of hats and make them their trade mark. Some people always wear long clothes and others only wear black and white.

As Diana Vreeland, the former editor of American *Vogue* said: 'Never worry about being vulgar, just worry about being boring.'

Learn to revamp your clothes so that they and you, look vaguely 'with it' and wildly individual. The latest accessories added to an old outfit can do wonders, or cut off the top of the extra length of a dress and turn the extra fabric into a scarf (which can be used on your head, around your waist or at your neck) or make it into a little purse – whatever is the look this year.

The best advice anyone can be given about fashion is to follow what Mme Girardin said: 'There is only one way to wear a beautiful dress: to forget you are wearing it.'

Self massage

The movements that you use when massaging someone else can equally easily be used on yourself. It isn't, obviously, going to be as pampering or as relaxing as *receiving* a massage, but it does mean that a massage is always available – at your finger tips! You will find that you can reach most areas to either stimulate or soothe. The movements you will use are stroking (effleurage), kneading (petrissage), pinching and pressures (pummelling).

Regular self massage can improve your circulation, alleviate tension and get rid of aches and pains. Also if you are feeling fat or flabby, stimulating massage can contribute to maintaining muscle tone, getting rid of ugly bulges and smoothing out 'bobbly' fat or cellulite, which so often appears when you have put on weight. In fact wherever you can reach – massage yourself.

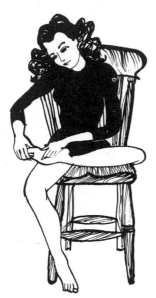

The feet

As I mention in *Zone therapy and Reflexology* (see page 143), it is thought that by massaging the foot you can stimulate the whole body. So if you have any aches and pains, try massaging the appropriate area of the foot. You may find it will help, and at the very least it will be marvellously relaxing. It is easy to reach your foot if you sit on a chair with your foot resting on your knee. So read the section on foot massage (page 97), and try it on yourself.

The leg

It is slightly more awkward massaging your own legs, especially the calves, but it is possible to stroke them upwards. If you've been doing too much sport the muscle in the calf can become very hard, and can ache; knead it from side to side, an alternating movement going from one side to the other.

Massage around the knee is surprisingly soothing – do rotaries all around the knee using your fingers and then cup and stroke around the knee with the palm of the hand.

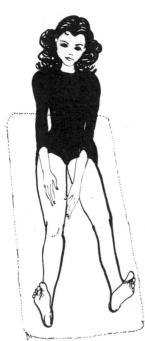

The thighs are probably the easiest place to massage yourself – which is lucky for all the thousands of women who suffer from slightly fat thighs. Knead and wring all over the thigh area remembering that you never drag the flesh down, always up. Imagine you are sculpting your body, and it will stay as you mould it, which is obviously in and up (wouldn't it be heavenly if it stayed like that?). But regular attention here, plus all the exercise, massage and good food I recommend, *will* make a visible difference.

The stomach

Stroke your tummy going in a clockwise direction around the colon. If you have a bit of excess fat on the tummy you can quite easily pinch and squeeze it, using the thumb and forefinger. Pinch and squeeze all over the diaphragm, stomach and hips. Finish by stroking.

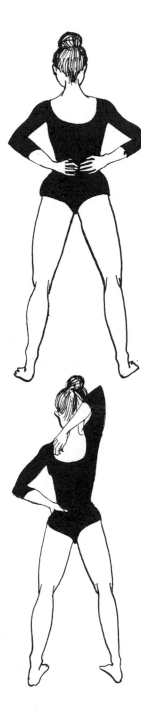

The hips and bottom
Stimulate these problem areas by stroking hard, kneading, wringing and pummelling.

The hands and arms
It is quite easy to massage your own hands. Do as much of the massage as you can manage (see page 105).

Stroke up the arm, from the hand to the shoulder. Knead all the way up. Do this by picking up the flesh and squeezing with one hand. Knead and pinch the upper arm. Really stimulate the circulation here as this area is often forgotten, and especially after winter can look less than glamorous with goose flesh and little spots. Massage will help to alleviate these problems, and so will scrubbing with a strong loofah or string glove (see page 69 for instructions on making your own string glove). Also check the Diet section as Vitamin A can help this condition.

The back
Unfortunately it really is not very easy to give yourself a satisfactory back massage – you'll just have to persuade a friend to learn the back massage on page 88 and practise on each other. But if your back is aching and no one is available, here are some movements that you can manage.

Using your fingers, do pressures and rotaries on either side of the spine, starting at the base and working up as high as possible.

Work around the shoulders. Using one hand at a time, working on the opposite shoulder, knead and pinch around the fleshy shoulder area.

Then do rotaries up the neck using the fingertips of both hands. Do these firm rotary pressures around the shoulder blade, in towards the spine and then on either side of the spine up the neck to the base of the skull.

'From birth to age 18 a girl needs good parents. From 18 to 35 she needs good looks. From 35–55 she needs good personality. From 55 on she needs good cash.'

Sophie Tucker

Getting fit

Each of us wants to be fit – to have the boundless energy of a really healthy body. Rather like a well-serviced car, a fit body runs more smoothly and without effort.

Everyone will have a different method for becoming fit – it might be through exercises, through yoga or tennis, weight-lifting, football, swimming or jogging. It really doesn't matter, as it is the end result we are interested in – a feeling of well-being and vitality, the readiness to tackle anything.

Many people have the mistaken idea that a toned-up muscle should be hard and taut, in other words muscle-bound. A really well-toned muscle should feel soft and elastic. A muscle in a state of readiness should be relaxed, not in a state of tension. Watch a cat, it lies around languidly but then suddenly leaps onto a table – there is no strain involved, it all looks effortless.

Watch other people doing any form of physical activity. Notice the ones who are obviously trying too hard. Their faces are screwed up, they are grimacing, sweating and pushing themselves to the limit. That can't be fun, and it all looks so strained and unpleasant.

Now look at someone who is at ease with their body. Watch an African running and you will see what I mean. The muscles are relaxed, the movements easy, with everything working in coordination, and it looks effortless.

I think that it is this relaxed effortlessness we need to remember when doing any form of exercise. So often I hear of people who rush into something, and are madly enthusiastic for a week. Thereafter they exhaust themselves (and their friends), it all fizzles out, and they are back in their unfit routine. It is better to go at it slowly, doing as much as you can with comfort, and slowly you will become fitter. It probably took you years to become unfit, and so you really cannot expect to become fit again in two days. Too much, too quick, and you will probably end up doing nothing at all. Again, a little does you good, whereas a lot may be unnecessary.

Tennis stimulates the circulation and burns up the calories. Serving stretches the waist and the running firms you up.

Swimming is especially good for overall toning and the back.

Running and bicycling are good for the legs.

Jogging. As with everything else you have to learn to jog. You will not get much benefit from sweating and straining and trotting along on flat feet. That will only exhaust you, and might even jar your spine and hurt your ankles.

I have heard of many people who have hurt themselves by rushing into jogging. If you are unfit and your muscles are suddenly overtaxed, the lack of blood may not only effect the extremities (cramp in the feet, for instance) but also the heart itself. I even heard of a man who died from a heart attack whilst jogging. I really am not trying to put you off jogging, just pointing out that as with every other form of physical activity you need to start off gently. Gradually as you become fit, you will find that you feel marvellous. You will feel more energetic, your body will become more lithe, and your complexion will improve.

Start by walking and gradually increase your speed until you are jogging along easily at about 5 m.p.h. At first only jog for about 10–15 minutes and then as you become fitter go for longer. Always start and finish by doing some stretching exercises (see page 147).

Avicenna (980–1037 AD) wrote much about the importance of exercise. He defined mild exercise *as 'swinging in a sitting, standing or lying position, horse riding, camel riding, elephant riding or carriage riding'. And* strenuous exercise, *according to his definition, includes 'wrestling, trials of strength against each other, running, brisk walking, hopping on one foot, fighting one's shadow with a spear or sword in hand until tired, skipping or restraining a fast running horse by pulling at the reins'.*

'Better to hunt in fields, for health unbought,
Than fee the doctor for a nauseous draught.
The wise, for cure, on exercise depend;
God never made his work, for man to mend.'

Epistles, To John Driden of Chesterton, Dryden

MEASUREMENT CHART

Beginning

Neck

Upper Arm

Chest/Bust

Wrist

Navel

Tummy
(2" below navel)

Hips

Bottom
(at largest point)

Upper Thigh

Mid Thigh

1" Above Knee

Calf

Ankle

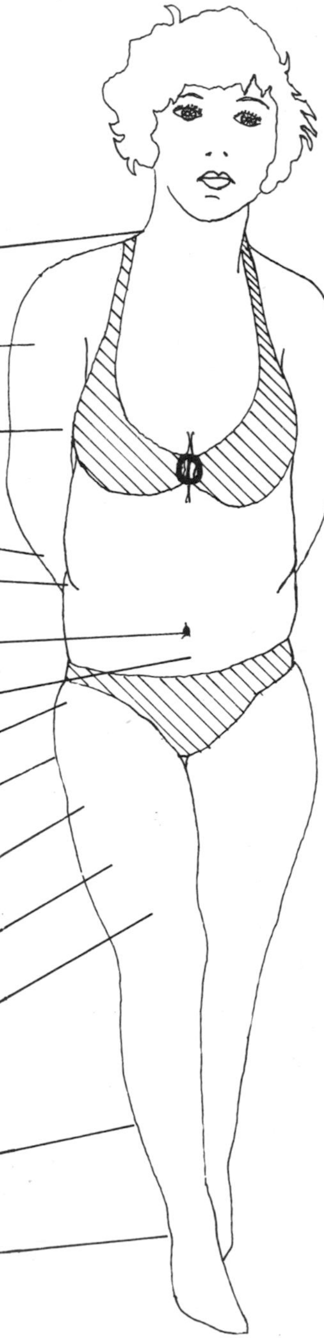

End of 1st Week

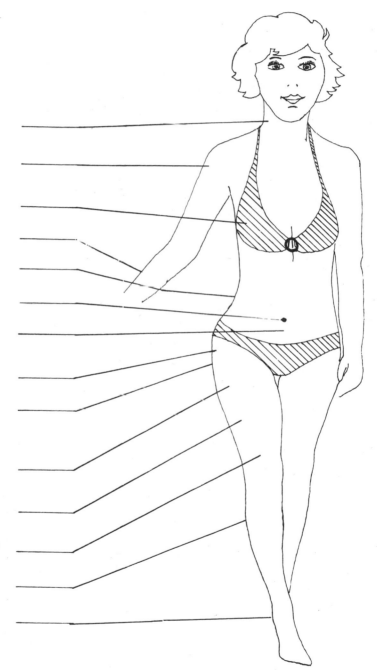

Neck

Upper Arm

Chest/Bust

Wrist

Navel

Tummy
(2" below navel)

Hips

Bottom
(at largest point)

Upper Thigh

Mid Thigh

1" Above Knee

Calf

Ankle

THE MIRROR TEST
WEIGHTS & MEASUREMENTS CHART

MY GOAL	WEIGHT	BUST	UPPER ARM	WAIST	MEASUREMENTS HIPS	THIGH	CALF	ANKLE
(I can write this in ink!)								
First Day								
Second Day								
Third Day								
Fourth Day								
Fifth Day								
Sixth Day								
Seventh Day								
Beginning of Second Week								
End of Second Week								
Beginning of Third Week								
End of Third Week								

MY GOOD POINTS
AREAS FOR SOME IMPROVEMENT
AREAS FOR DRASTIC IMPROVEMENT

(Do please fill in these charts – you can always rub out your pencil marks. You will be able to watch your progress over the two days, seven days or twenty one days – which can be so encouraging.)

HOW TO WORK OUT
YOUR IDEAL FIGURE

No two people have exactly the same figure, and that is why charts with the ideal weight for your height must always be an approximation.

However, it is possible to work out what your ideal measurements should be.

Carefully measure your left wrist and then by multiplying that you can calculate what all your other measurements should, ideally, be.

Bust	=	(wrist measurement)	×	6
Chest	=	(wrist measurement)	×	$5\frac{1}{2}$
Waist	=	(wrist measurement)	×	$4\frac{1}{2}$
Hips	=	(wrist measurement)	×	6
Thigh	=	(wrist measurement)	×	$3\frac{1}{2}$
Calf	=	(wrist measurement)	×	$2\frac{1}{4}$
Ankle	=	(wrist measurement)	×	$1\frac{1}{2}$

'It's a sort of bloom on a woman. If you have it [*charm*]*, you don't need to have anything else; and if you don't have it, it doesn't much matter what else you have.'*

What Every Woman Knows, Sir J. M. Barrie

Notes on Quantities

The following rough equivalents have proved useful to me:

60 drops	1 teaspoon
3 teaspoons	1 tablespoon
2 tablespoons	$\frac{1}{8}$ cup = 1 fl. oz.
4 tablespoons	$\frac{1}{4}$ cup = 2 fl. oz.
8 tablespoons	$\frac{1}{2}$ cup = 4 fl. oz.
12 tablespoons	$\frac{3}{4}$ cup = 6 fl. oz.
16 tablespoons	1 cup = 8 fl. oz.
32 tablespoons	2 cups = 16 fl. oz.

Since volume and weight are different measurements it is not possible to render the one in terms of the other in a simple table of equivalents, because bulk and weight do not correspond for all substances. In the case of oil, in fact, the same oil of different grades may have different weights.

60 drops	5 ml = 1 teaspoon
1000 mls	1 litre
1 litre	1.759 pints
1 pint	20 fl. oz. = 0.568 litres

weights

15.4 grains	1 gm.
28.3 gms	1 oz.
16 ozs	1 lb.
1 lb.	0.453 kilograms.
1 kilogram.	2.20 lbs

Recommended Reading

de Bairacli, Levy, Juliette: *The Herbal Handbook For Everyone,* Faber, 1966. Full of useful information, and yet easy to read.

Beard, Gertrude, and **Wood, Elizabeth:** *Massage Principles and Techniques,* Saunders and Co., 1964. A thorough guide to the history and movements of massage.

British Medical Association: *More Secret Remedies: What They Cost and What They Contain,* 1912. This shows how far we have managed to get away from what our grandmothers had to put up with.

Cameron, Allan: *Food – Facts and Fallacies,* Faber, 1971. Helps to develop a common-sense attitude towards the subject of food and nutrition.

Clark, Linda: *Secrets of Health and Beauty,* Pyramid Books, 1970. Lots of interesting ideas and facts on nutrition, health and home-made cosmetics.

Davies, Adèlle: *Let's Eat Right to Keep Fit,* Harcourt Brace Jovanovich, 1954. One of my favourite works on nutrition.

Downing, George: *The Massage Book,* Penguin, 1974. A clear guide to massage.

Enquire Within: Foulsham and Co. Ltd (various dates). Marvellously entertaining information on everything you want to know in your domestic, social or business life.

Freeman, Margaret: *Herbs for the Medieval Household,* The Metropolitan Museum of Art, New York, 1943. Odd snippets of information about herbs.

Grieve, Mrs M., FRHS: *A Modern Herbal,* Jonathan Cape, 1974. A comprehensive herbal, packed with facts. Both very interesting and highly readable.

Kirschmann, John D.: *Nutrition Almanac,* McGraw-Hill, Inc, 1973. A detailed study of nutrition.

de Langre, Jacques: *Do-In,* Happiness Press, 1971. Shows you how to do pressure point massage on yourself.

Light, Sidney, MD: *Massage, Manipulation and Traction*, Elizabeth Licht, 1960. A fascinating collection of papers on various methods of massage.

Ministry of Agriculture, Fishers and Food: *Manual of Nutrition*, Her Majesty's Stationery Office, London, 1977. A simple guide.

Morehouse, Lawrence, and **Gross, Leonard:** *Total Fitness in 30 Minutes a Week*, Mayflower, 1977. Tells how easy it is – or should be – to become and to remain fit.

Namikoshi, Tokujiro: *Shiatsu*, Japan Publications, 1975. I find this the best book on Shiatsu, and the easiest to follow.

Rose, Jeanne: *Herbal Body Book*, Grosset and Dunlap, 1976. Full of interesting ideas on the use of herbs and cosmetics.

Royce, Joyce: *Surface Anatomy*, F. A. Davis Co., Philadelphia, 1965. The beautiful photographs help to give one an understanding of the human body.

Rutledge, Deborah: *Natural Beauty Secrets*, Hawthorne Books, 1966. Full of amusing anecdotes and useful recipes.

Traven, Beatrice: *Here's Egg on Your Face*, Hewitt House, 1970. Full of cosmetic recipes which actually work; an ideal book.

Williams, Dr Roger: *Nutrition Against Disease*, Bantam Books, 1973. A fascinating study.

Yudkin, John: *This Slimming Business*, Penguin, 1962. A marvellously simply, straightforward book on low-carbohydrate slimming.

Yudkin, John: *Pure, White and Deadly*, Davis-Poynter Ltd, 1972. All about the horrors of eating too much sugar.

'Beauty – The power by which a woman charms her lover and terrifies her husband.'

The Devil's Dictionary, Ambrose Bierce

Index